THE *Skinny*
LOW CALORIE
RECIPE BOOK

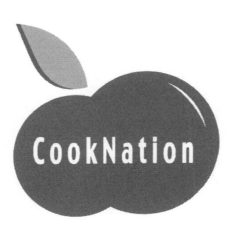

CookNation

The Skinny Low Calorie Meal Recipe Book
Great Tasting, Simple & Healthy Meals Under 300, 400 & 500 Calories. Perfect For Any Calorie Controlled Diet.

A Bell & Mackenzie Publication.
First published in 2014 by Bell & Mackenzie Publishing Limited.

ISBN 978-1-909855-51-9
A CIP catalogue record of this book is available from the British Library

Disclaimer
Some recipes may contain nuts or traces of nuts. Those suffering from any allergies associated with nuts should avoid any recipes containing nuts or nut based oils.

This information is provided and sold with the knowledge that the publisher and author do not offer any legal or other professional advice.

In the case of a need for any such expertise consult with the appropriate professional. This book does not contain all information available on the subject, and other sources of recipes are available.

This book has not been created to be specific to any individual's requirements.

Every effort has been made to make this book as accurate as possible. However, there may be typographical and or content errors. Therefore, this book should serve only as a general guide and not as the ultimate source of subject information.

This book contains information that might be dated and is intended only to educate and entertain.

The author and publisher shall have no liability or responsibility to any person or entity regarding any loss or damage incurred, or alleged to have incurred, directly or indirectly, by the information contained in this book.

Contents

Introduction   7

Low Calorie Breakfasts   **11**
Balsamic Garlic & Rosemary Tomatoes   12
Mustard Mushrooms On Granary   13
Cajun Spinach Eggs   14
Berry Smoothie   15
Blue Cheese Omelette   16
Mango & Avocado Breakfast Salad   17
Scrambled Vegetable Omelette   18
Parmesan & Roasted Pepper Frittata   19
Victorian Breakfast   20
Eggs & Mushrooms   21

Low Calorie Lunches   **23**
Napolitano Spaghetti   24
Flaked Salmon Fillet & Savoy Cabbage   25
Dolcelatte Chicken Salad   26
Veggie Couscous   27
Anchovy & Garlic Spaghettini   28
Fresh Pea & Prawn Noodles   29
Broccoli & Chicken Stir-fry   30
Coriander Chicken & Rice   31
Chinese Pak Choi & Prawns   32
Peppers & Steak   33
Tuna Steak & Spiced Courgettes   34
Oregano & Chilli Spaghetti   35

Contents

Porcini & Thyme Linguine 36
Prawn & Chorizo Angel Hair Pasta 37
Cod, Asparagus & Avocado 38
Pan Fried Lemon & Paprika Haddock 39
Creamy Leek & Potato Soup 40
Horseradish Mackerel & Spinach 41
Broccoli & Cauliflower Soup 42
Chilli Prawns & Mango 43
Parmesan Crusted Salmon 44
Mushroom & Caramelised Onion Soup 45
Chicken Noodle Ramen 46
Fresh Asparagus & Watercress Soup 47
Lemon & Basil Zucchini Gnocchi 48
Penne, Peas & Beans 49
Warm Cucumber Tuna Salad 50
Avocado & Prawn Cocktail 51
Almond & Onion Sprout Salad 52
Prawn & Paprika Rice 53
Fresh Salad Broth 54
Asparagus & Portabella Open Sandwich 55
Sicilian Caponata 56
Cod & Olives In Tomato Sauce 57

Low Calorie Dinners **59**
Steak & Stilton Sauce 60
Chicken, Raisins & Rice 61
Spinach, Prawns & Pinenuts 62

Contents

Thai Pork Kebabs & Lime Couscous   63
Lamb Kheema Ghotala   64
Chicken & Olive Citrus Couscous   65
Steak & Dressed Greens   66
Chicken & Wilted Lettuce In Oyster Sauce   67
Sesame Veggie Noodles   68
Chicken Chow Mein   69
Pork, Pineapple & Peppers   70
Hoisin & Cashew Chicken Stir-fry   71
Chicken & Noodle Broth   72
Balsamic Steak & Rice Stir-fry   73
Lemongrass Chicken Thai Curry   74
Egg Molee   75
Spicy Lamb & Carrot Burger   76
Lemon & Olive Penne   77
Creamy Parma Pasta   78
Asian Chicken Salad   79
Chicken & Broccoli Linguine   80
Scallop Sauce Spaghetti   81
Salmon & Spanish Rice   82
Nepali Tuna Supper   83
Venison Kebabs & Yoghurt   84
Lime & Thyme Squid Noodles   85
Mustard Haddock Chowder   86
Watercress Gnocchi   87
Jamaican Chicken Salad   88
Sweet & Spicy Steak Salad   89

Contents

Lemon & Oregano Tuna Steaks   90

Pea & Parmesan Risotto   91

Greek Chicken Kebabs   92

Cavalfiori Risotto   93

Fennel & Chickpea Chicken   94

Minted Fish Couscous   95

Other CookNation Titles   **97**

Introduction

Making Every Calorie Count

You may be following a specific diet or just want to make every calorie count, either way you will find each of our skinny low calorie recipes delicious, healthy, simple to make and guilt free.

Filling breakfasts to kick-start your day, fuss-free lunches and flavour filled dinners for any day of the week all under 300, 400 and 500 calories.

A calorie-controlled diet needn't be a daily struggle of denying yourself what you really want. Choice and taste are still paramount when eating low calorie dishes and we've put together a wonderful selection of meals that are tasty and nutritious and most can be prepared and cooked in less than 30 minutes.

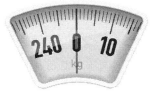

If you are counting your calories then it's safe to assume your goal is either to lose weight or maintain your current weight through a healthy and balanced eating plan and lifestyle.

Eating well can help you maintain or reduce your weight as well as cutting the risk of diabetes, high cholesterol and high blood pressure to name a few. Balancing plenty of fruit and vegetables, bread, rice, pasta and potatoes with protein-rich meat, fish, eggs, beans and dairy products are a good recipe for a healthy diet.

Calorie Control

It's important to remember what exactly a calorie is when controlling the number we consume.

A calorie is a unit of energy.

Scientifically, 1 calorie is the amount of energy required to raise one gram of water by one degree Celsius.

To you and I, a calorie (a unit of energy) is a vital component of our body and its health. We need energy to go about our every day tasks and for our body to function and repair itself as it should. So energy (calories) are a necessity and are present in everything we eat – carbohydrates, protein and fat. We know that excess calories are linked to weight gain and poor health so maintaining a healthy level of calories or reducing calories to accelerate weight loss should be managed carefully and safely.

Below is the recommended daily calorie intake in the UK to maintain your current weight.

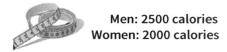 **Men: 2500 calories**
Women: 2000 calories

These figures can vary depending on your age and levels of physical activity.

It is also important to remember that maintaining your current weight involves balancing your calorie intake with the number of calories you burn through everyday activity. If your goal is to lose weight then you must burn more energy than the calories you are consuming.

Regular physical exercise combined with a healthy calorie controlled diet is the most effective way to manage your weight.

Our Skinny Recipes

All our recipes are simple and easy to follow and all fall below 300, 400 or 500 calories each. Many use low calorie and low fat alternatives to everyday products. We would encourage you to add these to your shopping basket each week and make a point of paying attention to food labeling whenever you can - some low fat products can be very high in sugar so watch out! Try switching to some of the following everyday items to keep calories and fat lower and be sure to take note of our kitchen essentials later in this chapter:

Low fat yogurt
Skimmed or semi skimmed milk
Reduced fat cheese
Low fat/unsaturated 'butter' spreads
Low fat crème fraiche
Low cal cooking oil spray
Low fat mayonnaise
Low fat single cream

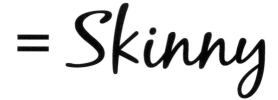

Ways To Cook

The methods we use to cook can also have a marked influence on the number of calories in a meal. Try adopting these healthier ways of cooking – you might be surprised how much better your food tastes!

Grilling
Although some foods such as white fish or chicken may require a light brushing of oil, often grilling requires no additional oil at all - red meats and oily fish are particularly suited to this method of cooking. Grilling can also achieve a crispy effect.

Stir-fry

By cooking quickly over a high heat with only a small amount of oil, much less fat is consumed – much healthier than deep or shallow frying.

Slow cooking

A great way to make a wholesome flavour-intense meal. By trimming meat of visible fat, this can be a great low calorie time saving way to cook.

Poaching

Great for fish and no additional oil needed!

Steaming

Again no oil needed and steamed food has a wonderfully fresh flavour and texture and retains many nutrients lost in other cooking methods. Steaming works well for meat, fish and vegetables.

Baking

Baking food in an oven often does not require additional oil to cook. Try wrapping in tin foil with a little wine to keep juices intact.

Kitchen Essentials

All our skinny low calorie recipes use simple, easily obtainable, store cupboard ingredients. To maintain a healthy diet we recommend keeping your kitchen stocked up with many of the following essentials and plenty of fresh fruit, veg & lean meat too!

Tomato puree Tomato passata Mixed Tinned beans Lemon juice Lime juice Cider Vinegar Rice wine vinegar Thai fish sauce Pitted black olives Dried pasta Rice Couscous Gnocchi	Straight-to-wok noodles Chicken & vegetable stock Runny honey Dried fruit & nuts Fresh Garlic Fresh ginger Papirka Turmeric English & Dijon mustard Ground coriander Crushed chilli flakes Dried Italian herbs	Olive oil Balsamic vinegar Soy Sauce Worcestershire sauce Tinned tuna (in water not brine or oil) Fresh herbs – coriander, flat leaf parsley, basil, chives, oregano, mint Free range eggs Crushed sea salt Ground black pepper

About CookNation

CookNation is the leading publisher of innovative and practical recipe books for the modern, health-conscious cook.

CookNation titles bring together delicious, easy and practical recipes with their unique approach - easy and delicious, no-nonsense recipes - making cooking for diets and healthy eating fast, simple and fun.

With a range of #1 best-selling titles - from the innovative 'Skinny' calorie-counted series, to the 5:2 Diet Recipes collection - CookNation recipe books prove that 'Diet' can still mean 'Delicious'!

Turn to the end of this book to browse all CookNation's recipe books.

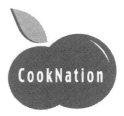

Skinny
LOW CALORIE
BREAKFASTS

Balsamic Garlic & Rosemary Tomatoes

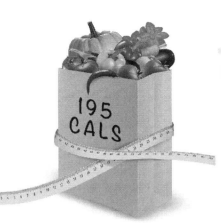

195 CALS

Ingredients   Serves 4

12 large beef tomatoes, quartered
4 garlic cloves, crushed
2 tsp dried rosemary
2 tbsp olive oil
1 tbsp balsamic vinegar

2 onions, sliced
2 small ciabatta rolls
Salt & pepper to taste

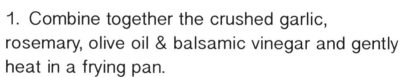

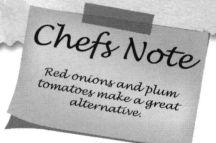

Chefs Note

Red onions and plum tomatoes make a great alternative.

1. Combine together the crushed garlic, rosemary, olive oil & balsamic vinegar and gently heat in a frying pan.

2. Season the tomatoes and saute in the frying pan along with the onions for 8-10 minutes or until the tomatoes are softened and cooked through.

3. Cut the ciabatta rolls in half and lightly toast. Pile the balsamic onions and tomatoes on top of the ciabatta halves and serve.

Mustard Mushrooms On Granary

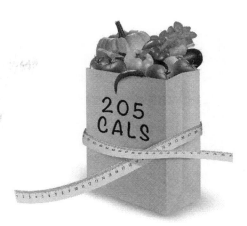

205 CALS

Ingredients   Serves 4

1 tbsp olive oil
2 garlic cloves, crushed
1 onion, sliced
500g/1lb 2oz mushrooms, sliced
1 tbsp Dijon mustard

120ml/½ cup low fat crème fraiche
4 pieces granary bread, lightly toasted
2 tbsp freshly chopped flat leaf parsley
Salt & pepper to taste

Chefs Note

You could substitute English mustard in this recipe but it will be a lot 'hotter'!

1. Gently saute the onions and garlic in the olive oil for a few minutes. Add the mushrooms and continue cooking for 8-10 minutes or until the mushrooms are soft and cooked through.

2. Stir through the mustard and creme fraiche, combine well and warm through.

3. Pile the creamy mushrooms and onions onto the granary toast and sprinkle with chopped parsley.

4. Season and serve.

Cajun Spinach Eggs

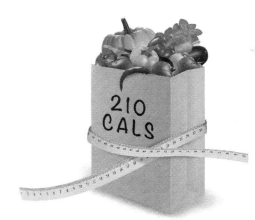

210 CALS

Ingredients Serves 4

2 red peppers, deseeded & sliced
1 tsp paprika
½ tsp each chilli powder, cumin, coriander & salt
8 large free-range eggs

1 tbsp olive oil
125g/4oz spinach leaves
Salt & pepper to taste

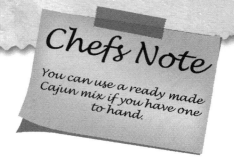

Chefs Note
You can use a ready made Cajun mix if you have one to hand.

1. Break the eggs into a bowl, add the dried spices & salt and lightly beat with a fork.

2. Gently heat the oil in a frying pan and add the peppers.

3. Saute for a few minutes until they begin to soften.

4. Add the spinach and allow to wilt for a minute or two. Pour in the beaten eggs and move around the pan until the eggs begin to scramble. As soon as they start to set remove from the heat and serve with lots of black pepper.

Berry Smoothie

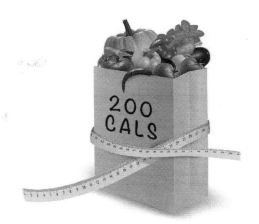

200 CALS

Ingredients   Serves 4

200g/7oz blueberries
300g/11oz strawberries
2 large ripe bananas

500ml/2 cups fat free Greek yogurt
2 tsp runny honey

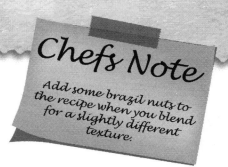

Chefs Note

Add some brazil nuts to the recipe when you blend for a slightly different texture.

1. Remove the strawberry stalks and peel the bananas.

2. Blend all the ingredients together. Check the sweetness of the smoothie and add a little more honey if needed.

3. Divide into 4 glasses and serve immediately.

Blue Cheese Omelette

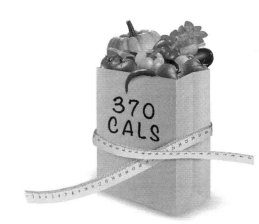

370 CALS

Ingredients   Serves 1

2 large free-range eggs
40g/1½oz stilton cheese, crumbled
1 tsp olive oil

50g/2oz watercress
Salt & pepper to taste

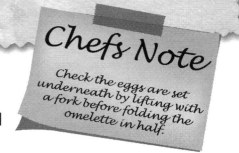

Chefs Note

Check the eggs are set underneath by lifting with a fork before folding the omelette in half.

1. Lightly beat the eggs with a fork. Season well and add the crumbled blue cheese.

2. Gently heat the oil in a small frying pan and add the omelette mixture. Tilt the pan to ensure the mixture is evenly spread over the base.

3. Cook on a low to medium heat and, when the eggs are set underneath, fold the omelette in half and continue to cook for a further 2 minutes.

4. Serve with the watercress sprinkled all over the top.

Mango & Avocado Breakfast Salad

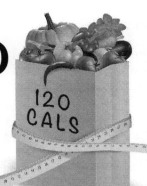

Ingredients   Serves 4

2 ripe avocados, peeled, stoned & cubed

1 ripe mango, peeled, stoned & cubed

250g/9oz plum tomatoes, diced

½ tsp paprika

1 red onion, finely chopped

½ red chilli, deseeded & finely chopped

2 tbsp lime juice

1 tbsp freshly chopped coriander

150g/5oz watercress or rocket leaves

Salt & pepper to taste

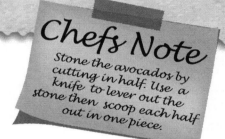

Chefs Note
Stone the avocados by cutting in half. Use a knife to lever out the stone then scoop each half out in one piece.

1. Combine the cubed avocado, mango, tomatoes, paprika, onions, chilli, lime & coriander together. Allow to sit for a few minutes to let the flavour infuse.

2. Pile onto a bed of watercress or rocket leaves, season & serve.

Scrambled Vegetable Omelette

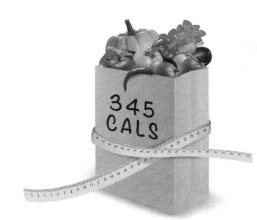

Ingredients   Serves 4

400g/14oz baby new potatoes, halved
125g/4oz tenderstem broccoli, roughly chopped
1 tbsp olive oil

1 onion, sliced
1 tsp turmeric & paprika
½ tsp chilli powder
8 large free-range eggs
Salt & pepper to taste

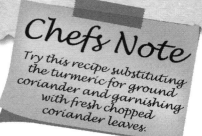

Chefs Note

Try this recipe substituting the turmeric for ground coriander and garnishing with fresh chopped coriander leaves.

1. Place the potatoes and chopped broccoli in salted boiling water. Boil for 4-6 minutes or until the potatoes are tender. Drain and put to one side.

2. Meanwhile gently heat the olive oil in a frying pan and saute the onions for a few minutes until softened. Add the potatoes, broccoli & dried spices to the pan and stir. Cook for a minute or two longer before adding the eggs to the pan.

3. Increase the heat and cook until the eggs are scrambled. Check the seasoning & serve immediately.

Parmesan & Roasted Pepper Frittata

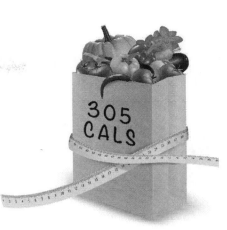

305 CALS

Ingredients   Serves 4

1 tbsp olive oil
1 onion, chopped
125g/4oz courgettes, sliced
250g/9oz roasted peppers, drained & chopped

10 free-range eggs
1 tbsp grated Parmesan cheese
2 tbsp freshly chopped flat leaf parsley
Salt & pepper to taste

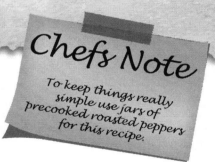

Chefs Note

To keep things really simple use jars of precooked roasted peppers for this recipe.

1. Heat the oil in a frying pan and gently saute the onions and courgettes for a few minutes until softened. Add the peppers and continue to cook for 2-3 minutes longer.

2. Break the eggs into a bowl and combine with Parmesan cheese. Tip the softened onions and courgettes into the bowl. Mix well and return the eggs & vegetables to the pan, tilting to ensure the mixture covers the base evenly.

3. Cover the pan, reduce the heat and leave to cook for a few minutes. Flip the frittata over and cook the other side until the eggs set and the vegetables are tender.

4. Cut into wedges and serve with chopped parsley sprinkled over the top.

Victorian Breakfast

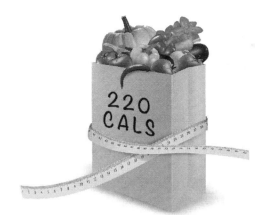

220 CALS

Ingredients   Serves 4

8 fresh lambs' kidneys
1 tbsp olive oil
4 garlic cloves, crushed
75g/3oz button mushrooms, halved
1 onion, sliced
2 tbsp Worcestershire sauce

1 tsp cayenne pepper
120ml/½ cup low fat crème fraiche
75g/3oz spinach leaves
2 English breakfast muffins, lightly toasted
Salt & pepper to taste

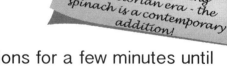

Chefs Note
Lambs' kidneys are a traditional breakfast often served during the Victorian era - the spinach is a contemporary addition!

1. Prepare the lambs' kidneys by cutting in half and trimming out any tough core.

2. Gently saute the garlic, mushrooms & onions for a few minutes until softened.

3. Add the kidneys, Worcestershire sauce and cayenne pepper to the pan. Combine well and cook the kidneys for approx. 4-5 minutes each side.

4. When the kidneys are cooked through, stir in the creme fraiche and spinach and warm through.

5. Season and serve on the toasted English muffins.

Eggs & Mushrooms

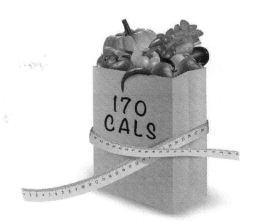

170 CALS

Ingredients   Serves 4

8 tsp low fat soft cheese
2 tbsp freshly chopped chives
2 garlic cloves, crushed
8 large flat mushrooms
4 large free-range eggs

1 handful rocket leaves
Salt & pepper to taste

Chefs Note
You can buy low fat soft cheese with chives already added.

1. Preheat the oven grill.

2. Mix the soft cheese, chives & garlic together and spread evenly on the underside of each mushroom. Season well and place, underside up, under the grill for 5-7 minutes or until the mushrooms are cooked through.

3. Meanwhile fill a frying pan with boiling water and break the eggs into the gently simmering pan to poach while the mushrooms cook.

4. Put the mushrooms on the plates. Arrange the rocket over the top and add a poached egg.

5. Serve with lots of black pepper.

Skinny
LOW CALORIE
LUNCHES

Napolitano Spaghetti

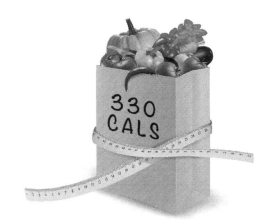

330 CALS

Ingredients   Serves 4

300g/11oz dried spaghetti
2 tbsp olive oil
400g/14oz cherry tomatoes, roughly chopped
200g/7oz pitted black olives, roughly chopped
2 stalks celery, finely chopped
1 onion, finely chopped

3 garlic cloves, crushed
1 tbsp tomato puree
4 tbsp freshly chopped basil
Salt & pepper to taste

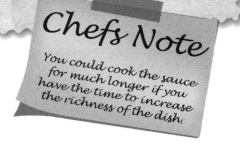

Chefs Note

You could cook the sauce for much longer if you have the time to increase the richness of the dish.

1. Heat the oil and gently saute the tomatoes, olives, celery, onions, garlic, tomato puree & basil for 10-15 minutes or until the tomatoes lose their shape and combine to make a sauce.

2. Whilst the sauce is cooking place the spaghetti in a pan of salted boiling water until tender. Drain the cooked pasta and add to the frying pan.

3. Toss well, season & serve.

Flaked Salmon Fillet & Savoy Cabbage

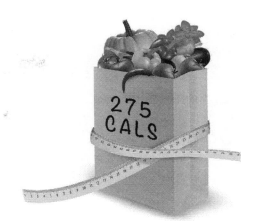

275 CALS

Ingredients   Serves 4

500g/1lb 2oz skinless salmon fillets
1 savoy cabbage, shredded
1 tbsp olive oil
2 garlic cloves, crushed
2 tbsp freshly chopped chives

2 tbsp low fat crème fraiche
2 tbsp horseradish sauce
2 tbsp lemon juice
Salt & pepper to taste

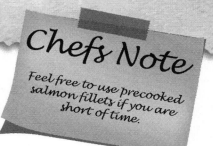

Chefs Note

Feel free to use precooked salmon fillets if you are short of time.

1. Season the salmon fillets and place under a preheated grill for 10-12 minutes or until cooked through. Flake and put to one side to cool.

2. Steam the cabbage for 8-10 minutes or until the cabbage is tender. Meanwhile heat the oil and garlic in a saucepan and gently saute for a minute or two. Add the cooked cabbage, stir well and cook for a minute or two longer.

3. Gently combine together the chives, creme fraiche, horseradish sauce, lemon juice & flaked salmon.

4. Divide the dressed salmon and sauteed cabbage onto plates, season & serve.

Dolcelatte Chicken Salad

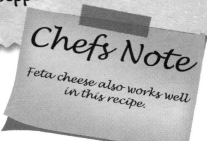

370 CALS

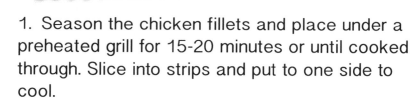

Ingredients   Serves 4

500g/1lb 2oz skinless chicken breast
200g/7oz cherry tomatoes
100g/3½oz Dolcelatte cheese
2 ripe avocados, peeled & stoned
2 tbsp extra virgin olive oil

2 tbsp cider vinegar
2 tbsp low fat crème fraiche
1 tsp paprika
300g/11oz watercress
Salt & pepper to taste

Chefs Note
Feta cheese also works well in this recipe.

1. Season the chicken fillets and place under a preheated grill for 15-20 minutes or until cooked through. Slice into strips and put to one side to cool.

2. Halve the cherry tomatoes and crumble the Dolcelatte cheese.

3. Combine together the olive oil, vinegar, creme fraiche & paprika to make a dressing.

4. Toss the dressing, tomatoes, cheese, avocados & watercress together in a large bowl.

5. Divide onto plates and arrange the chicken slices on top. Season and serve.

Veggie Couscous

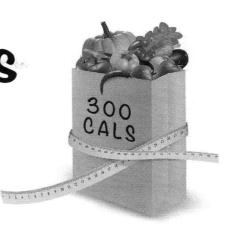

300 CALS

Ingredients   Serves 4

1 tbsp olive oil
2 courgettes, sliced
2 red peppers, deseeded & sliced
2 tbsp pitted black olives, chopped
1 onion, chopped
2 garlic cloves, crushed
1 tsp ground coriander

1 tbsp lemon juice
1½/370ml cups vegetable stock
200g/7oz couscous
2 tbsp sultanas, chopped
Lemon wedges to serve
2 tbsp freshly chopped coriander
Salt & pepper to taste

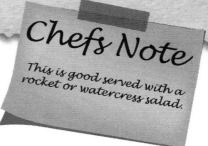

Chefs Note

This is good served with a rocket or watercress salad.

1. Gently saute the courgettes, peppers, olives, onions, garlic, ground coriander & lemon juice for a 7-10 minutes or until softened and cooked through.

2. Whilst the vegetables are cooking, place the couscous & sultanas is a pan with the hot stock. Bring the pan to the boil, remove from the heat, cover and leave to stand for 3-4 minutes or until all the stock is absorbed and the couscous is tender.

3. Fluff the couscous with a fork and pile into the pan with the cooked vegetables. Mix well, divide onto plates and serve with fresh lemon wedges on the side & chopped coriander sprinkled over the top.

Anchovy & Garlic Spaghettini

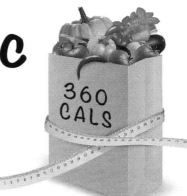

360 CALS

Ingredients   Serves 4

300g/11oz dried spaghettini
12 tinned anchovy fillets, drained
4 tbsp olive oil
4 garlic cloves, crushed
2 red onions, sliced

3 tbsp lemon juice
4 tbsp freshly chopped basil
Salt & pepper to taste

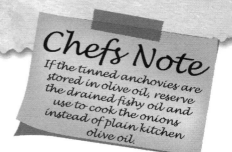

Chefs Note
If the tinned anchovies are stored in olive oil, reserve the drained fishy oil and use to cook the onions instead of plain kitchen olive oil.

1. Cook the pasta in a pan of salted boiling water until tender.

2. Place the anchovy fillets and oil in a high-sided frying pan and gently saute along with the garlic, red onions & lemon juice whilst the pasta cooks. After a little while the anchovy fillets should dissolve to make a salty sauce base.

3. When the pasta is tender, drain and add to the frying pan. Combine really well to make sure every strand spaghettini is covered with the oil and anchovy sauce.

4. Sprinkle with the freshly chopped basil. Season & serve.

Fresh Pea & Prawn Noodles

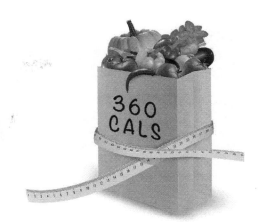

360 CALS

Ingredients   Serves 4

1 tbsp olive oil
4 garlic cloves, crushed
1 tbsp freshly grated ginger
½ tsp crushed chilli flakes
500g/1lb 2oz shelled, raw king prawns
1 onion, sliced
2 red peppers, deseeded & sliced

60ml/¼ cup soy sauce
2 tbsp Thai fish sauce
200g/7oz fresh peas
400g/14oz straight to wok noodles
Lemon wedges to serve
Salt & pepper to taste

Chefs Note

This simple stir-fry works equally well with sliced chicken breast.

1. Heat the olive oil in a frying pan and gently saute the garlic and ginger for a minute. Add the chilli flakes, prawns, onions, peppers, soy sauce, fish sauce & fresh peas and cook for 8-10 minutes or until the peppers soften and the prawns pink up.

2. Add the noodles and combine for 3-4 minutes or until the noodles are piping hot and the prawns are cooked through.

3. Season and serve with lemon wedges.

Broccoli & Chicken Stir-fry

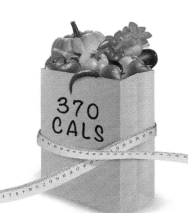

370 CALS

Ingredients   Serves 4

400g/14oz skinless chicken breast, sliced
400g/14oz tenderstem broccoli
1 tbsp olive oil
2 garlic cloves, crushed
1 onion, chopped

2 tbsp soy sauce
60ml/¼ cup chicken stock
200g/7oz spinach leaves, chopped
250g/9oz rice
Salt & pepper to taste

Chefs Note
As a time saver microwaveable rice is a handy store cupboard ingredient for quick stir-fry's.

1. Season the chicken and roughly chop the broccoli.

2. Place the rice in salted boiling water and cook until tender.

3. Meanwhile heat the olive oil in a frying pan and gently saute the garlic and onions for a few minutes.

4. Add the chicken & chopped broccoli to the pan along with the soy sauce and chicken stock. Stir-fry for 8-10 minutes until the chicken is cooked through.

5. Add the drained rice to the pan along with the spinach.

6. Combine for a minute or two, check the seasoning and serve.

Coriander Chicken & Rice

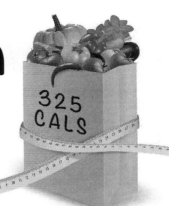

325 CALS

Ingredients   Serves 4

250g/9oz rice
2 tbsp coriander seeds
2 tbsp fenugreek seeds
1 tbsp olive oil
2 garlic cloves, crushed

1 red chilli, deseeded & finely chopped
400g/14oz skinless chicken breast, sliced
2 tbsp soy sauce
2 large free-range eggs
Salt & pepper to taste

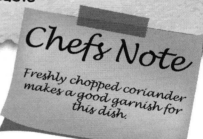

Chefs Note

Freshly chopped coriander makes a good garnish for this dish.

1. Place the rice in salted boiling water and cook until tender.

2. Meanwhile bash the coriander and fenugreek seeds with a pestle and mortar.

3. Heat the olive oil in a frying pan and gently saute the garlic for a minute along with the bashed seeds.

4. Add the chilli, chicken & soy sauce and cook for 5-10 minutes or until the chicken is cooked through.

5. Add the drained rice to the pan along with the eggs. Increase the heat, stir-fry for 3-4 minutes.

6. Season & serve.

Chinese Pak Choi & Prawns

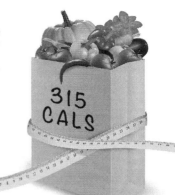

315 CALS

Ingredients Serves 4

250g/9oz rice
2 pak choi
60ml/¼ cup chicken stock
1 tbsp olive oil
2 garlic cloves, crushed
1 onion, sliced

1 tbsp freshly grated ginger
500g/1lb 2oz shelled raw king prawns
1 tbsp soy sauce
2 tsp Chinese five spice powder
1 tsp crushed chilli flakes
Salt & pepper to taste

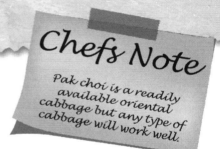

Chefs Note

Pak choi is a readily available oriental cabbage but any type of cabbage will work well.

1. Place the rice in salted boiling water and cook until tender.

2. Shred the pak choi and gently wilt in a frying pan with the chicken stock for a few minutes until tender.

3. Heat the olive oil in a frying pan and saute the garlic, onions & ginger for a minute or two.

4. Add the prawns, soy sauce, Chinese five spice powder & chilli flakes and cook until the prawns are pink. Check the prawns are cooked through.

5. Add the drained rice to the pan and combine for a minute or two.

6. Quickly toss through the pak choi. Season and serve immediately.

Peppers & Steak

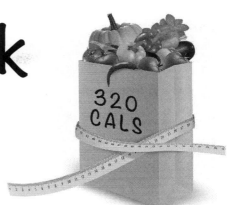

320 CALS

Ingredients   Serves 4

400g/14oz sirloin steak
2 tbsp olive oil
1 tsp paprika
1 onion, sliced
2 garlic cloves, crushed

4 red & yellow peppers, deseeded & sliced
400g/14oz cherry tomatoes
4 baby gem lettuces, shredded
50g/2oz feta cheese, crumbled
Salt & pepper to taste

1. Trim any fat off the steak. Lightly brush with a little of the olive oil & all the paprika. Season and put a frying pan on a high heat.

Chefs Note

You could choose to use Stilton cheese instead of feta for this lovely fresh recipe.

2. In another pan gently saute the peppers, onions & garlic in the rest of the olive oil for 5-7 minutes or until tender.

3. Place the steak in the smoking hot dry pan and cook for 1-2 minutes each side, or to your liking. Leave to rest for 3 minutes and then finely slice.

4. Halve the tomatoes & shred the lettuces. Add the peppers, crumble the feta cheese and combine on plates.

5. Place the sliced steak on top. Season and serve.

Tuna Steak & Spiced Courgettes

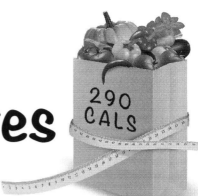

290 CALS

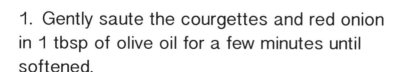

Ingredients   Serves 4

300g/11oz courgettes, diced
1 red onion, finely chopped
2 tbsp olive oil
4 fresh tuna steaks, each weighing
125g/4oz

6 tbsp balsamic vinegar
400g/14oz watercress
Salt & pepper to taste

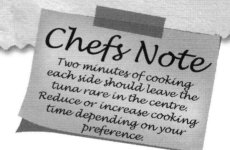

Chefs Note

Two minutes of cooking each side should leave the tuna rare in the centre. Reduce or increase cooking time depending on your preference.

1. Gently saute the courgettes and red onion in 1 tbsp of olive oil for a few minutes until softened.

2. Season the tuna and put a frying pan on a high heat with the rest of the olive oil and balsamic vinegar.

3. Place the tuna in the pan and cook for 2 minutes each side. Remove the tuna from the pan and serve with the watercress and courgette side dish.

Oregano & Chilli Spaghetti

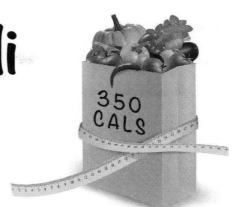

Ingredients   Serves 4

300g/11oz dried spaghetti
2 tsp dried oregano
½ tsp crushed chilli flakes
2 tbsp pitted black olives, chopped
1 onion, sliced

4 tbsp sundried tomato puree
2 tbsp olive oil
Salt & pepper to taste

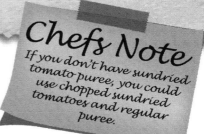

Chefs Note
If you don't have sundried tomato puree, you could use chopped sundried tomatoes and regular puree.

1. Cook the spaghetti in a pan of salted boiling water until tender.

2. Meanwhile gently saute the oregano, chilli, olives, onions & sundried tomato puree for a few minutes or until the onions are softened. Drain the cooked pasta and add to the pan.

3. Toss well, season & serve.

Porcini & Thyme Linguine

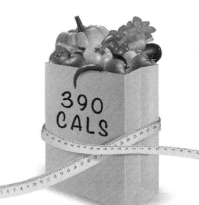

390 CALS

Ingredients   Serves 4

50g/2oz dried porcini mushrooms
300g/11oz dried linguine
1 tbsp olive oil
2 garlic cloves, crushed
1 onion, sliced

2 tsp dried thyme
2 tbsp low fat mascarpone cheese
1 tbsp tomato puree
Salt & pepper to taste

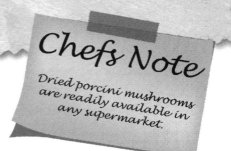

Chefs Note

Dried porcini mushrooms are readily available in any supermarket.

1. Place the porcini mushrooms in a little boiling water and leave to rehydrate for 10-15 minutes. Thinly slice when softened.

2. Cook the spaghetti in a pan of salted boiling water until tender.

3. Heat the olive oil in a high-sided frying pan and gently saute the garlic, onions & dried thyme whilst the pasta cooks.

4. When the onions are soft add the mascarpone cheese, and tomato puree and stir well. Drain the cooked pasta and add to the frying pan.

5. Toss well. Season & serve.

Prawn & Chorizo Angel Hair Pasta

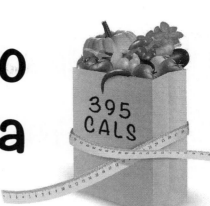

395 CALS

Ingredients   Serves 4

300g/11oz dried angel hair pasta
1 tbsp olive oil
2 garlic cloves, crushed
50g/2oz chorizo, finely chopped or sliced
1 tsp paprika
1 onion, sliced

250g/9oz shelled raw king prawns, chopped
4 tbsp lemon juice
4 tsp freshly chopped flat leaf parsley
Salt & pepper to taste

Chefs Note

Chorizo and shellfish are a classic combination. Serve with lots of freshly ground black pepper.

1. Cook the spaghetti in a pan of salted boiling water until tender.

2. Meanwhile heat the olive oil in a high-sided frying pan and gently saute the garlic, chorizo, paprika and onions for 5 minutes whilst the pasta cooks.

3. Add the chopped prawns and lemon juice and cook until the prawns are pink and cooked through. Drain the cooked pasta, add to the frying pan and combine really well.

4. Sprinkle with chopped parsley and serve.

Cod, Asparagus & Avocado

315 CALS

Ingredients
Serves 4

2 garlic cloves, crushed
2 tbsp olive oil
200g/7oz asparagus spears
4 boneless, skinless cod fillets each weighing 125g/4oz
250g/9oz ripe plum tomatoes, finely chopped
1 bunch spring onions, finely chopped
2 avocados, peeled & stoned
2 tbsp freshly chopped oregano
200g/7oz watercress
1 lime, cut into wedges
Salt & pepper to taste

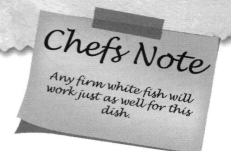

Chefs Note
Any firm white fish will work just as well for this dish.

1. Mix together the garlic & olive oil and brush onto the cod fillets & asparagus spears.

2. Place the fish and asparagus under a preheated grill and cook for 5-7 minutes or until the cod is cooked through and the asparagus spears are tender

3. Meanwhile combine the chopped tomatoes, spring onions, avocados, chopped oregano & watercress together.

4. Season and serve the cooked cod with the watercress tomato salad & lime wedges.

Pan Fried Lemon & Paprika Haddock

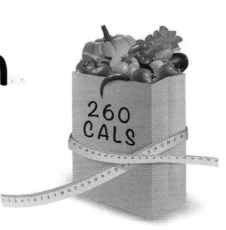

260 CALS

Ingredients   Serves 4

4 boneless, skinless haddock fillets each weighing 125g/4oz
1 onion, sliced
200g/7oz mushrooms
1 tsp each paprika & mixed spice

3 tbsp lemon juice
2 tbsp olive oil
150g/5oz rocket
Salt & pepper to taste

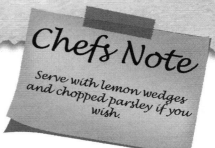

Chefs Note
Serve with lemon wedges and chopped parsley if you wish.

1. Season the haddock fillets.

2. Gently saute the garlic in the olive oil for a few minutes. Add the onions, mushrooms, paprika, mixed spice & lemon juice and cook for 5-8 minutes or until the onions are softened.

3. Move the vegetables to one side of the pan to make room for the haddock fillets. Cook for 3-5 minutes each side depending on the thickness of the fillet, or until cooked through.

4. Serve the cooked haddock fillets on a bed of rocket with the onions & mushrooms arranged over the top of the fish.

Creamy Leek & Potato Soup

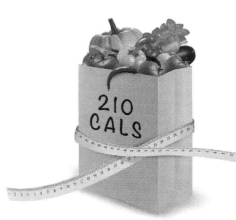

210 CALS

Ingredients   Serves 4

500g/1lb 2oz potatoes
500g/1lb 2oz leeks
1lt/4 cups vegetable stock/broth

60ml/¼ cup low fat single cream
Salt & pepper to taste

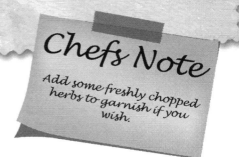

Chefs Note

Add some freshly chopped herbs to garnish if you wish.

1. Peel and chop the potatoes & leeks.

2. Place the potatoes and leeks in a saucepan
with the hot stock. Bring to the boil and leave to simmer for 10-12 minutes or until the potatoes and tender.

3. Blend the soup to a smooth consistency, stir through the cream, check the seasoning and serve.

Horseradish Mackerel & Spinach

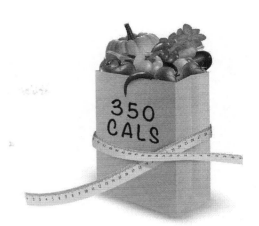

350 CALS

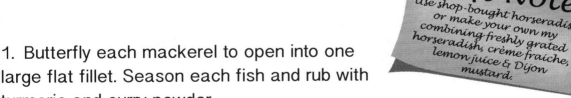

Ingredients   Serves 4

4 fresh, boned headless mackerel each weighing 150g/5oz
1 tsp turmeric
2 tsp curry powder
1 tbsp olive oil
2 tbsp horseradish sauce

1 tbsp lemon juice
2 tbsp chopped capers
300g/11oz spinach
Salt & pepper to taste

Chefs Note

Use shop-bought horseradish or make your own my combining freshly grated horseradish, crème fraiche, lemon juice & Dijon mustard.

1. Butterfly each mackerel to open into one large flat fillet. Season each fish and rub with turmeric and curry powder.

2. Heat the olive oil in a pan and fry the mackerel for 3 minutes each side.

3. Meanwhile combine together the horseradish sauce, lemon juice & capers to make a dressing.

4. When the fish is cooked, wrap in foil and put to one side to keep warm. Add the spinach to the empty pan and cook for a few minutes. Stir the dressing through the wilted spinach and serve with the cooked mackerel fillets.

Broccoli & Cauliflower Soup

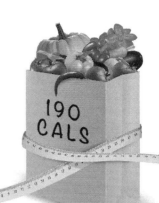

190 CALS

Ingredients   Serves 4

200g/7oz cauliflower florets, chopped

200g/7oz broccoli florets, chopped

75g/3oz potatoes, peeled & chopped

1 onion, chopped

1 tsp ground coriander

1lt/4 cups vegetable stock/broth

250ml/1 cup semi skimmed milk

Salt & pepper to taste

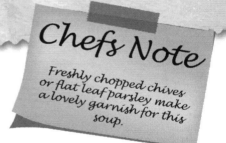

Chefs Note

Freshly chopped chives or flat leaf parsley make a lovely garnish for this soup.

1. Add all the ingredients, except the milk, to the saucepan.

2. Bring to the boil and leave to simmer for 10-12 minutes or until the vegetables are tender.

3. Blend to a smooth consistency, add the milk, and heat through for a minute or two. Check the seasoning and serve.

Chilli Prawns & Mango

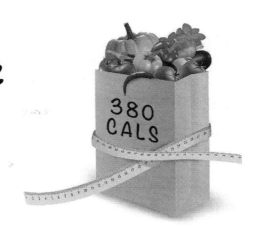

380 CALS

Ingredients
Serves 4

250g/9oz rice
1 red pepper, deseeded & sliced
1 onion, sliced
2 garlic cloves, crushed
1 tbsp freshly grated ginger
½ tsp brown sugar

1 tbsp olive oil
1 tbsp soy sauce
500g/1lb 2oz shelled raw king prawns
1 tsp dried chilli flakes
1 mango, stoned & finely chopped
4 tbsp freshly chopped coriander
2 tbsp lime juice
Salt & pepper

Chefs Note

Reduce the amount of crushed chillies in the dish if you don't want the meal to have too much 'kick'.

1. Place the rice in salted boiling water and cook until tender.

2. Gently saute the sliced peppers, onions, garlic, ginger & sugar in the olive oil for a few minutes until softened.

3. Add the prawns & chilli flakes and cook for 5-8 minutes or until the prawns are pink and cooked through.

4. Add the drained rice to the pan, combine well and cook together for a minute or two longer.

5. Combine together the mango, coriander and lime juice to make a mango salsa.

6. Divide the prawns and rice into bowls and serve with the mango salsa piled on top.

Parmesan Crusted Salmon

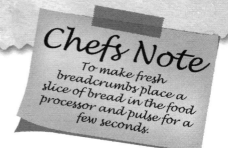

390 CALS

Ingredients   Serves 4

500g/1lb 2oz baby new potatoes, halved

4 boneless, skinless salmon fillets each weighing 125g/4oz

2 tbsp grated Parmesan cheese

3 tbsp fresh breadcrumbs

2 garlic cloves, crushed

200g/7oz tenderstem broccoli

Lemon wedges to serve

Salt & pepper to taste

Chefs Note
To make fresh breadcrumbs place a slice of bread in the food processor and pulse for a few seconds.

1. Cook the new potatoes in a pan of salted boiling water until tender.

2. Meanwhile season the salmon fillets. Mix the Parmesan cheese, breadcrumbs & garlic together and coat the top of the salmon fillets with the breadcrumb mixture.

3. Place the salmon under a preheated grill and cook for 10-13 minutes or until the salmon fillets are cooked through.

4. Whilst the salmon and potatoes are cooking plunge the broccoli into salted boiling water and cook for a 2-3 minutes or until tender.

5. Drain the potatoes and broccoli and serve with the salmon fillets and lemon wedges.

Mushroom & Caramelised Onion Soup

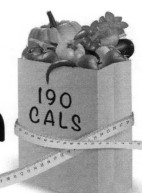

190 CALS

Ingredients   Serves 4

1 tsp olive oil
2 garlic cloves, crushed
2 onions, chopped
2 tbsp balsamic vinegar
200g/7oz potatoes, peeled & diced

500g/1lb 2oz mushrooms, sliced
1ltml/4 cups vegetable stock/broth
Salt & pepper to taste

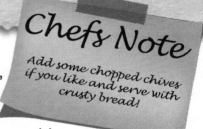

Chefs Note
Add some chopped chives if you like and serve with crusty bread!

1. Heat the oil in a saucepan and add the garlic, onions & balsamic vinegar. Saute on a high heat until the onions are cooked crispy brown and the balsamic vinegar reduces down. Put to one side when caramelised.

2. Meanwhile add the potatoes, mushrooms & stock to a saucepan. Bring to the boil and simmer for 8-10 minutes or until the potatoes are soft.

3. Blend to a smooth consistency and divide into bowls.

4. Split the onions equally and place in the centre of each bowl of soup. Season and serve.

Chicken Noodle Ramen

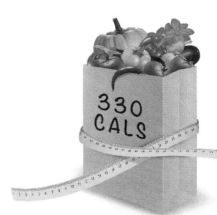

330 CALS

Ingredients · Serves 4

- 2 leeks, sliced
- 2 celery stalks, chopped
- 2 carrots, chopped
- 1 tsp dried thyme
- 1lt / 4 cups chicken stock
- 1 bunch spring onions, sliced thinly lengthways
- 250g/9oz cooked chicken breast, shredded
- 200g/7oz tinned sweetcorn, drained
- 400g/14oz straight to wok ramen noodles
- Salt & pepper to taste

Chefs Note

Dried noodles are fine to use too. Just use half the quantity and cook for a little longer in the stock.

1. Place the leeks, celery and carrots in a saucepan along with the thyme and stock. Bring to the boil and simmer for 7-10 minutes or until all the vegetables are soft.

2. Blend to a smooth consistency and return to the pan. Add the shredded chicken, sweetcorn & noodles and cook for a further 4-6 minutes or until the ramen is piping hot.

3. Check the seasoning and serve with the sliced spring onions on top.

Fresh Asparagus & Watercress Soup

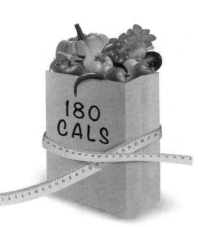

180 CALS

Ingredients Serves 4

125g/4oz potatoes, finely chopped
1 tbsp olive oil
2 garlic cloves, crushed
1 tsp dried thyme
1 onion, sliced
750ml/3 cups vegetable stock/broth

400g/14oz asparagus tips
250ml/1 cup dry white wine
150g/5oz watercress
Salt & pepper to taste

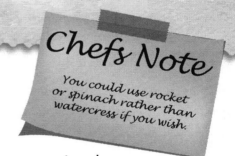

Chefs Note

You could use rocket or spinach rather than watercress if you wish.

1. Add all the ingredients, except the watercress, to a saucepan. Bring to the boil and simmer for 5-7 minutes, or until the potatoes are tender.

2. Roughly blend the soup with just a couple of pulses in the food processor. Stir through the watercress, check the seasoning and serve immediately.

Lemon & Basil Zucchini Gnocchi

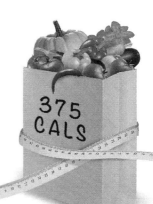

375 CALS

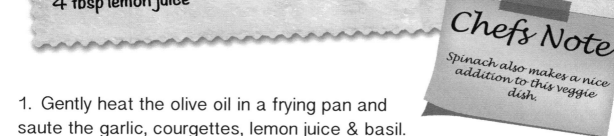

Ingredients   Serves 4

3 tbsp olive oil
2 garlic cloves, crushed
300g/11oz baby courgettes, thinly sliced lengthways
4 tbsp lemon juice

4 tbsp freshly chopped basil
700g/1lb 9oz gnocchi
Salt & pepper to taste

Chefs Note

Spinach also makes a nice addition to this veggie dish.

1. Gently heat the olive oil in a frying pan and saute the garlic, courgettes, lemon juice & basil.

2. Meanwhile place the gnocchi in a pan of salted boiling water. Cook for 2-3 minutes or until the gnocchi begins to float to the top. As soon as the gnocchi is cooked, drain and place in the frying pan with the courgettes on a high heat.

3. Move the gnocchi around for a minute or two to coat each dumpling in oil. Season and serve.

Penne, Peas & Beans

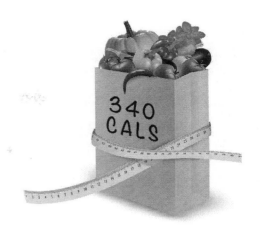

340 CALS

Ingredients   Serves 4

150g/5oz baby broad beans
300g/11oz dried penne
1 tbsp olive oil
2 garlic cloves, crushed
150g/5oz fresh peas

120ml/½ cup low fat crème fraiche
2 tbsp freshly chopped mint
Salt & pepper to taste

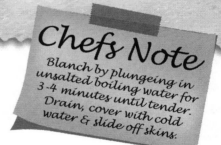

Chefs Note
Blanch by plungeing in unsalted boiling water for 3-4 minutes until tender. Drain, cover with cold water & slide off skins.

1. Blanch the broad beans and remove the skins.

2. Cook the penne in a pan of salted boiling water until tender.

3. Meanwhile gently heat the olive oil in a high-sided frying pan and saute the blanched broad beans, garlic & peas whilst the pasta cooks. When the peas and beans are cooked through stir in the creme fraiche and mint.

4. Drain the cooked penne and add to the pan.

5. Toss well, season & serve with lots of freshly ground black pepper.

Warm Cucumber Tuna Salad

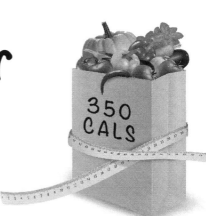

350 CALS

Ingredients   Serves 4

1 cucumber, finely sliced into matchsticks
2 tsp caster sugar
120ml/½ cup rice wine vinegar
½ tsp dried chilli flakes
1 red onion, finely chopped
400g/14oz tinned tuna, drained

400g/14oz tinned borlotti beans, drained & rinsed
125g/4oz cherry tomatoes, halved
200g/7oz rocket
Salt & pepper to taste

Chefs Note

This is a simple Asian salad. You may need to balance the sugar and vinegar a little.

1. Place the cucumber in a frying pan and gently warm over a low heat. Add the caster sugar, rice wine vinegar & chilli flakes. Simmer for a few minutes and set aside to cool.

2. Meanwhile mix together the red onion, beans, tomatoes & tuna in a large bowl. Add the cooled cucumber, toss with the rocket and serve.

Avocado & Prawn Cocktail

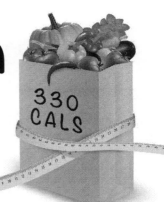

330 CALS

Ingredients
Serves 4

2 tbsp low fat mayonnaise
2 tbsp low fat crème fraiche
2 tsp tomato ketchup
1 dash tobasco sauce
1 tbsp lemon juice
2 tbsp freshly chopped chives

500g/1lb 2oz cooked & peeled prawns
2 Romaine lettuces, shredded
2 ripe avocados, peeled, stoned & diced
1 cucumber, diced
1 tsp cayenne pepper
Salt & pepper to taste

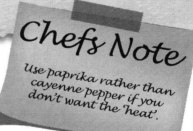

Chefs Note

Use paprika rather than cayenne pepper if you don't want the 'heat'.

1. Mix together the mayonnaise, creme fraiche, ketchup, tobasco sauce, lemon juice, chives & prawns until everything is really well combined.

2. In a separate bowl gently combine the shredded lettuce, avocado & cucumber to make a salad.

3. Divide the salad on four plates and pile the dressed prawns on top

4. Sprinkle with cayenne pepper and serve.

Almond & Onion Sprout Salad

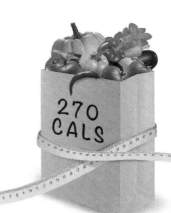

270 CALS

Ingredients   Serves 4

500g/1lb 2oz prepared Brussels sprouts
3 tbsp olive oil

2 onions, sliced
150g/5oz blanched almonds
Salt & pepper to taste

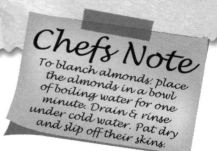

Chefs Note
To blanch almonds: place the almonds in a bowl of boiling water for one minute. Drain & rinse under cold water. Pat dry and slip off their skins.

1. Slice the sprouts really thinly so they fall into shreds.

2. Heat the olive oil in a frying pan and gently saute the onions for 8-10 minutes or until they are soft and golden.

3. Meanwhile plunge the shredded sprouts into salted boiling water for 2 minutes. Drain and rinse through with cold water. Add to the onion pan along with the almonds and toss until piping hot and cooked through.

4. Season with plenty of salt & freshly ground pepper to serve.

Prawn & Paprika Rice

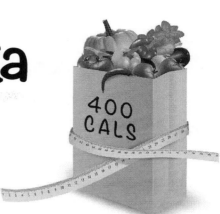

400 CALS

Ingredients   Serves 4

1 tbsp olive oil
2 garlic cloves, crushed
1 onion, sliced
2 red peppers, deseeded & sliced
300g/11oz cherry tomatoes, halved

250g/9oz rice
1 tbsp paprika
400g/14oz peeled raw prawns
Salt & pepper to taste

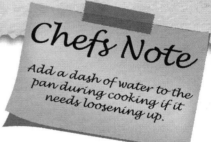

Chefs Note

Add a dash of water to the pan during cooking if it needs loosening up.

1. Heat the olive oil in a frying pan and gently saute the garlic, onions, peppers & tomatoes for 15-20 minutes or until everything is softened and forms a combined base.

2. Meanwhile place the rice in salted boiling water and cook until tender.

3. Add the prawns & paprika to the frying pan and cook until piping hot and cooked through.

4. When the rice is ready, drain and add to the pan.

5. Toss well. Season and serve.

Fresh Salad Broth

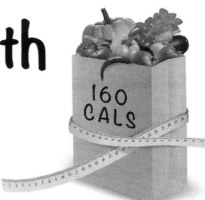

160 CALS

Ingredients   Serves 4

1 tbsp olive oil
1 garlic clove, crushed
1 onion, sliced
1 carrot, diced
150g/5oz potatoes, peeled & diced
2 tsp dried mixed herbs

1lt/4 cups chicken or
vegetable stock
150g/5oz watercress,
roughly chopped
Salt & pepper to taste

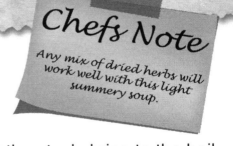

Chefs Note

Any mix of dried herbs will work well with this light summery soup.

1. Heat the olive oil in a pan and gently saute the garlic, sliced onions, carrots, potatoes & dried herbs for a few minutes until softened. Add the stock, bring to the boil, cover and leave to simmer for 10-15 minutes or until everything is tender.

2. Blend to your preferred consistency and add the watercress.

3. Stir through, season and serve immediately.

Asparagus & Portabella Open Sandwich

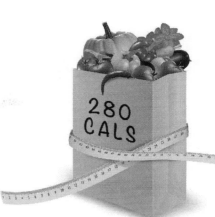

280 CALS

Ingredients
Serves 4

2 tbsp olive oil
20 asparagus spears, chopped
4 large portabella mushrooms, sliced
1 onion, sliced
1 tsp dried basil

3 tbsp lemon juice
½ tsp crushed chilli flakes
2 tbsp freshly chopped flat leaf parsley
2 ciabatta rolls
Salt & pepper to taste

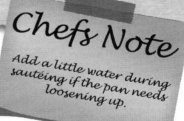

Chefs Note
Add a little water during sautéing if the pan needs loosening up.

1. Heat the olive oil in a pan and gently saute the asparagus, mushrooms, onions & basil for a few minutes until softened.

2. Meanwhile spilt the ciabatta rolls in half and gently toast.

3. When the mushrooms and asparagus are tender add the lemon juice and chilli flakes. Stir through, season and serve on top of each ciabatta half with the chopped parsley sprinkled on top.

Sicilian Caponata

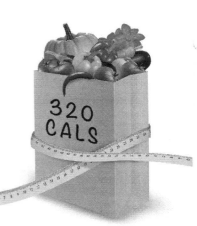

320 CALS

Ingredients   Serves 4

1 tbsp olive oil
2 aubergines, cubed
200g/7oz baby courgettes, sliced in half lengthways
1 tsp dried oregano
2 onions, sliced
1 celery stalk, chopped
2 garlic cloves, crushed
3 tbsp balsamic vinegar
1 tbsp capers, chopped
200g/7oz ripe plum tomatoes, roughly chopped
2 tbsp pitted black olives, sliced
2 tbsp sultanas, roughly chopped
200g/7oz rice
Salt & pepper to taste

Chefs Note

Caponata is a southern Italian dish which can also be served cold!

1. Gently saute the aubergines, courgettes, oregano, onions, celery and garlic in the olive oil for a few minutes until softened. Add the balsamic vinegar, capers, tomatoes, olives & sultanas and continue to cook for 20-25 minutes or until everything is cooked through and tender.

2. Whilst the aubergines are cooking place the rice in salted boiling water and cook until tender.

3. Add the drained rice to the pan. Combine well, season & serve.

Cod & Olives In Tomato Sauce

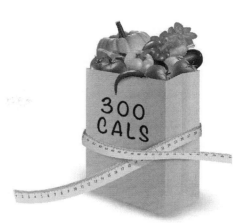

300 CALS

Ingredients   Serves 4

1 tbsp olive oil
½ red chilli, deseeded & finely sliced
1 onion, sliced
2 garlic cloves, crushed
200g/7oz ripe plum tomatoes,
roughly chopped

2 tbsp sundried tomato puree
4 tbsp pitted green olives, sliced
600g/1lb 5oz skinless, boneless cod
fillets
2 tbsp freshly chopped flat leaf parsley
Salt & pepper to taste

Chefs Note
This is even better served with a slice of fresh crusty bread to mop up all the lovely tomato juices.

1. Gently saute the onion, chilli and garlic in the olive oil for a few minutes until softened. Add the chopped tomatoes, puree & olives and leave to gently simmer for 10 minutes stirring occasionally.

2. Season the fish fillets and cut into thick slices. Add the fish to the pan and combine well. Cover and leave to gently simmer for 10-15 minutes or until the fish is cooked through and piping hot. Sprinkle with chopped parsley and serve.

Skinny
LOW CALORIE
DINNERS

Steak & Stilton Sauce

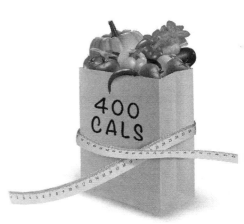

Ingredients   Serves 4

500g/1lb 2oz sweet potatoes
4 sirloin steaks each weighing
125g/4oz
1 tbsp olive oil
200g/7oz fresh peas

75g/3oz stilton cheese
3 tbsp crème fraiche
120ml/½ cup chicken stock
Salt & pepper to taste

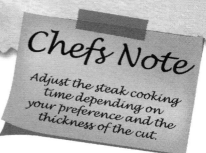

Chefs Note

Adjust the steak cooking time depending on your preference and the thickness of the cut.

1. Peel the sweet potatoes, cut into 1cm slices and cook in the saucepan for 10-12 minutes or until they are tender.

2. Meanwhile trim any fat off the steak. Season and brush with the olive oil while you put a frying pan on a high heat.

3. Place the steak in the smoking hot dry pan and cook for 1-2 minutes each side, or to your liking. When the steak is cooked put to one side to rest for 3 minutes.

4. Whilst the steak is resting quickly cook the peas in salted boiling water for a minute or two. In a separate pan gently heat and stir the stilton, creme fraiche and stock to make a sauce.

5. Serve the steak, sweet potatoes & fresh peas with the stilton sauce drizzled over the top.

Chicken, Raisins & Rice

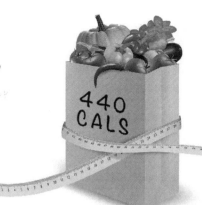

440 CALS

Ingredients Serves 4

250g/9oz rice
1 tbsp olive oil
3 garlic cloves, crushed
1 onion, chopped
200g/7oz raisins

500g/1lb 2oz skinless chicken breast, diced
4 beef tomatoes, toughly chopped
4 tbsp freshly chopped coriander
Salt & pepper to taste

1. Place the rice in a pan of salted boiling water and cook until tender.

2. Heat the oil in a frying pan and gently saute the onions & garlic for a few minutes until softened.

Chefs Note

Feel free to toss the coriander through the dish rather than serving as a garnish if you prefer.

3. Add the raisins, chicken & chopped tomatoes and continue to cook until the chicken is cooked through.

4. When the chicken is cooked through add the drained rice to the pan and combine.

5. Remove from the heat, stir well and serve with chopped coriander sprinkled over the top.

Spinach, Prawns & Pinenuts

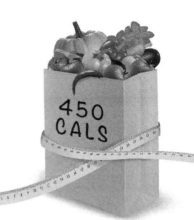

450 CALS

Ingredients   Serves 4

250g/9oz rice
1 tbsp olive oil
1 onion, chopped
1 tbsp freshly grated ginger
1 green chilli, deseeded & finely sliced
2 garlic cloves, crushed

2 tbsp lime juice
400g/14oz raw, peeled king prawns
200g/7oz spinach
120ml/ ½ cup chicken stock
3 tbsp pine nuts
Salt & pepper to taste

Chefs Note
If you have time, gently toast the pinenuts in a dry pan for a couple of minutes until golden brown.

1. Place the rice in a pan of salted boiling water and cook until tender.

2. Heat the olive oil in a frying pan and gently saute the onions, garlic, sliced chilli & ginger for a few minutes until softened.

3. Add the lime juice, prawns, spinach & stock and cook for 5-8 minutes on a high heat until the stock has reduced and the prawns are cooked through.

4. Tip the drained rice into the pan along with pinenuts.

5. Remove from the heat, stir well, season & serve.

Thai Pork Kebabs & Lime Couscous

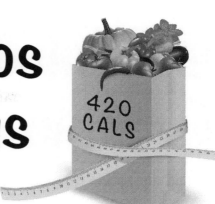

420 CALS

Ingredients   Serves 4

500g/1lb 2oz pork tenderloin, cubed
1 tbsp Thai green curry paste
1 tbsp coconut cream
1 tbsp soy sauce
1 lime cut into 8 wedges
2 onions, cut into 8 wedges each

370ml/1½ cups chicken stock
200g/7oz couscous
2 tbsp lime juice
8 kebab sticks
Lemon wedges to serve
Salt & pepper to taste

Chefs Note
You can use any combination of vegetables you prefer with the pork to make the kebabs.

1. Season the pork and preheat the grill.

2. Mix together the curry paste, coconut cream & soy sauce. Add the cubed pork and combine well.

3. Place the pork, lime wedges and onion wedges in turn on the skewers, put under the grill and cook for 10-13 minutes or until the pork is cooked through.

4. Whilst the pork is cooking, place the couscous in a pan with the hot stock and lime juice. Bring the pan to the boil, remove from the heat, cover and leave to stand for 3-4 minutes or until all the stock is absorbed and the couscous is tender.

5. Fluff the couscous with a fork, divide onto plates and serve with the pork kebabs.

Lamb Kheema Ghotala

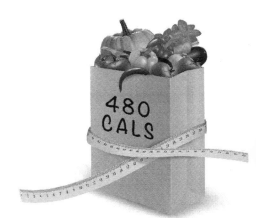

480 CALS

Ingredients   Serves 4

200g/7oz rice
2 tbsp olive oil
2 onions, sliced
3 garlic cloves, crushed
2 large beef tomatoes, roughly chopped

2 tbsp curry powder
400g/14oz lean lamb mince
4 free range eggs
Salt & pepper to taste

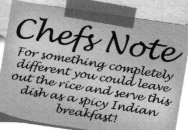

Chefs Note

For something completely different you could leave out the rice and serve this dish as a spicy Indian breakfast!

1. Place the rice in a pan of salted boiling water and cook until tender.

2. Meanwhile heat the oil in a frying pan and gently saute the onions & garlic for a few minutes until softened.

3. Add the tomatoes, curry powder and mince to the pan. Increase the heat and brown for 2-3 minutes.

4. Reduce the heat, stir well and cook for 6-10 minutes or until the mince is cooked through.

5. Whilst the rice is cooking break the eggs. Lightly beat with a fork and add to the lamb mince. Stir though to scramble for a minute or two.

6. Add the drained rice and combine well. Season and serve.

Chicken & Olive Citrus Couscous

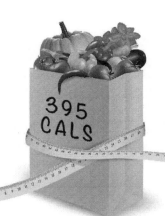

395 CALS

Ingredients
Serves 4

500g/1lb 2oz skinless chicken breast, diced
1 tbsp olive oil
1 red pepper, deseeded & finely chopped
4 tbsp black pitted olives, sliced
2 garlic cloves, crushed

1 onion, sliced
370ml/1½ cups chicken stock
200g/7oz couscous
1 orange, juice & zest
1 lemon, juice & zest
Salt & pepper to taste

1. Season the chicken.

2. Gently saute the peppers, olives, garlic and onions in the olive oil for a few minutes until softened. Add the chicken to the pan and cook for 6-8 minutes or until cooked through.

3. Whilst the chicken is cooking place the couscous in a saucepan with the hot stock. Bring the pan to the boil, remove from the heat, cover and leave to stand for 3-4 minutes or until all the stock is absorbed and the couscous is tender.

4. Fluff the couscous with a fork and add to the frying pan along with the orange & lemon juice & zest.

5. Toss really well and serve immediately.

Chefs Note

Some freshly chopped mint makes a great addition to this dish.

Steak & Dressed Greens

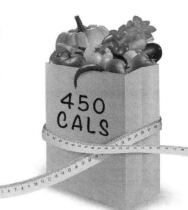

450 CALS

Ingredients   Serves 4

500g/1lb 2oz mini salad potatoes, quartered
4 sirloin steaks, each weighing 125g/4oz
250g/9oz spring greens

1 tbsp olive oil
1 tsp runny honey
1 orange, zest & juice
Salt & pepper to taste

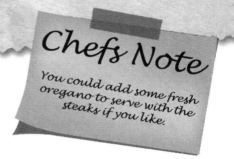

Chefs Note

You could add some fresh oregano to serve with the steaks if you like.

1. Place the potatoes and spring greens into a saucepan of salted water and cook for 6-8 minutes or until tender.

2. Trim any fat off the steak, season and lightly brush with olive oil. Place the steak in a smoking-hot pan and cook for 1-2 minutes each side, or to your liking. When the steak is cooked, put to one side to rest for 3 minutes.

3. Combine together the olive oil, honey, orange juice & zest to make a dressing.

4. Drain the potatoes and greens and place in a bowl with the dressing. Season and combine well.

5. Serve the steak with the dressed potatoes & greens on the side.

Chicken & Wilted Lettuce In Oyster Sauce

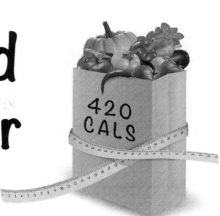

420 CALS

Ingredients
Serves 4

250g/9oz rice
1 tbsp olive oil
2 red peppers, deseeded & sliced
200g/7oz mushrooms, sliced
500g/1lb 2oz skinless chicken
breasts, chopped
5 tbsp oyster sauce
2 iceberg lettuces, shredded
Salt & pepper to taste

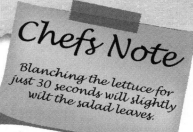

Chefs Note
Blanching the lettuce for just 30 seconds will slightly wilt the salad leaves.

1. Place the rice in a pan of salted boiling water and cook until tender.

2. Heat the olive oil in a frying pan or wok and gently saute the peppers and mushrooms for a few minutes until softened.

3. Add the chicken and oyster sauce to the pan and fry on a high heat for 4-5 minutes or until the chicken is cooked through.

4. At the end of this cooking time plunge the shredded lettuce into salted boiling water for 30 seconds.

5. Add the drained rice to the pan and toss together. Season and serve immediately on top of the blanched lettuce.

Sesame Veggie Noodles

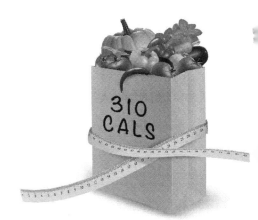

310 CALS

Ingredients   Serves 4

1 tbsp fish sauce
1 tbsp sesame oil
4 tbsp soy sauce
2 tbsp lime juice
2 tsp runny honey
2 tsp sesame seeds

2 red chillies, deseeded & finely chopped
4 tbsp freshly chopped coriander
600g/1lb 5oz straight-to-wok egg noodles
Salt & pepper to taste

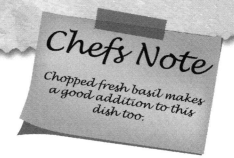

Chefs Note

Chopped fresh basil makes a good addition to this dish too.

1. Mix together the fish sauce, sesame oil, soy sauce, lime juice, honey, sesame seeds & chillies to make a dressing.

2. Gently warm the dressing in a saucepan and add the noodles. Cook for a few minutes until the noodles are piping hot. Divide into shallow bowls, sprinkle with chopped coriander, season & serve.

Chicken Chow Mein

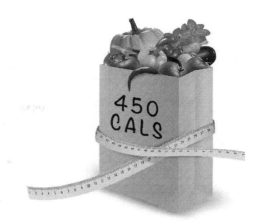

450 CALS

Ingredients

Serves 4

400g/14oz skinless chicken breasts
1 tsp Chinese 5 spice powder
1 tbsp olive oil
2 garlic cloves, crushed
2 carrots, cut into match sticks
1 onion, sliced
1 pointed cabbage, shredded

2 tbsp rice wine vinegar
1 tbsp fish sauce
3 tbsp sweet chilli sauce
1 tbsp soy sauce
250g/9oz beansprouts
600g/1lb 5oz straight-to-wok egg noodles
Salt & pepper

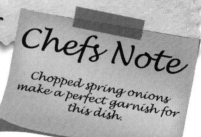

Chefs Note

Chopped spring onions make a perfect garnish for this dish.

1. Slice the chicken breast and mix with the 5 spice powder.

2. Heat the olive oil in a deep sided frying pan and gently saute the garlic, carrots and onions for a few minutes until softened.

3. Add the chicken and cabbage to the pan and cook for 5-7 minutes or until the chicken is cooked through.

4. Mix together the rice wine vinegar, fish sauce, sweet chilli sauce and soy sauce together to make a combined sauce. Add the beansprouts, noodles & sauce to the pan and cook until the dish is piping hot.

5. Divide into shallow bowls, season & serve.

Pork, Pineapple & Peppers

425 CALS

Ingredients   Serves 4

1 tbsp olive oil
2 yellow peppers, deseeded & sliced
1 onion, sliced
1 red chilli, deseeded & finely chopped
400g/14oz pork tenderloin, diced
200g/7oz pineapple chunks, drained
and chopped
120ml/½ cup pineapple juice
2 tbsp soy sauce
4 tbsp lime juice
600g/1lb 5oz straight-to-wok egg noodles
1 tbsp freshly chopped flat leaf parsley
Salt & pepper to taste

Chefs Note

Prawns are a good alternative to pork in this recipe.

1. Heat the olive oil in a frying pan or wok and gently saute the peppers, onions and chopped chilli for a few minutes until softened.

2. Add the pork, pineapple juice, pineapple chunks, soy sauce & lime juice and continue to stir-fry until the pork is cooked through.

3. Add the noodles to the pan and cook until piping hot. Divide into shallow bowls, sprinkle with chopped parsley & serve.

Hoisin & Cashew Chicken Stir-fry

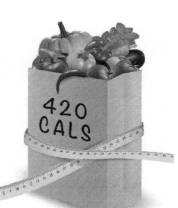

420 CALS

Ingredients   Serves 4

250g/9oz rice
400g/14oz skinless chicken breast
1 tsp runny honey
1 tbsp olive oil
1 onion, chopped
2 red peppers, deseeded & sliced
200g/7oz mangetout, trimmed

100g/3½oz baby sweetcorn, chopped
1 pak choi, shredded
125g/4oz cashew nuts, halved
2 tbsp soy sauce
1 tsp cornflour
2 tbsp hoisin sauce
Salt & pepper to taste

Chefs Note

Feel free to substitute other vegetables in place of mangetout and baby corn.

1. Place the rice in a pan of salted boiling water and cook until tender.

2. Cube the chicken and mix with the honey.

3. Heat the olive oil in a frying pan or wok and gently saute the chopped onions, peppers, mangetout & sweetcorn for a few minutes until softened.

4. Add the chicken, pak choi & nuts to the pan and cook for 4-5 minutes or until the chicken is cooked through.

5. Mix together the soy sauce, cornflour and hoisin sauce to make a smooth paste (add a little water if needed). Add to the pan, turn up the heat and cook until the dish is piping hot and the chicken is cooked through..

6. Add the drained rice to the pan. Combine well, season and serve immediately.

Chicken & Noodle Broth

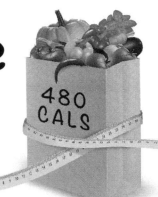

480 CALS

Ingredients   Serves 4

200g/7oz peas
2 garlic cloves, crushed
1lt/4 cups chicken stock
1 tbsp freshly grated ginger
4 tbsp soy sauce
150g/5oz spinach, chopped

600g/1lb 5oz straight-to-wok egg noodles
400g/14oz cooked chicken breast, shredded
2 tbsp coconut cream
1 bunch spring onions, chopped
Salt & pepper to taste

Chefs Note
Using cooked chicken means you can shred the meat finely before adding to the pan, which benefits the texture of the broth.

1. Place all the ingredients, except the chicken, coconut cream and spring onions, in a sauce pan.

2. Gently cook for a 5-7 minutes. Add the shredded chicken and coconut cream, combine well and keep on the heat until the chicken is piping hot.

3. Divide into four bowls and serve with the chopped spring onions sprinkled over the top.

Balsamic Steak & Rice Stir-fry

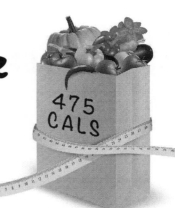

475 CALS

Ingredients   Serves 4

250g/9oz rice
1 tbsp olive oil
1 red pepper, deseeded & finely sliced
1 onion, sliced
200g/7oz asparagus tips
200g/7oz baby sweetcorn, sliced lengthways

2 garlic cloves, crushed
2 carrots, cut into fine matchsticks
500g/1lb 2oz sirloin steak, thinly sliced
1 tbsp soy sauce
2 tsp runny honey
3 tbsp balsamic vinegar
Salt & pepper to taste

Chefs Note
Trim the steak of any visible fat before slicing.

1. Place the rice in a pan of salted boiling water and cook until tender.

2. Heat the oil in a frying pan or wok and gently saute the red peppers, onions, garlic cloves, asparagus tips, baby corn and carrots for a few minutes until softened.

3. Add the steak, soy sauce, honey and balsamic vinegar and cook on a high heat for 1-2 minutes.

4. Add the drained rice to the pan and combine well. Season and serve.

Lemongrass Chicken Thai Curry

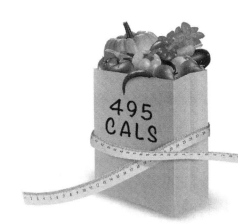

495 CALS

Ingredients   Serves 4

400g/14oz skinless, chicken breast
1 tbsp olive oil
1 onion, sliced
1 stalk lemongrass, finely chopped
1 tsp brown sugar
1 tbsp Thai green curry paste
2 tbsp lime juice
1 tbsp soy sauce
250ml/1 cup chicken stock
250ml/1 cup low fat coconut milk
600g/1lb 5oz straight-to-wok egg noodles
75g/3oz watercress
Salt & pepper to taste

Chefs Note

Red Thai curry paste works just as well in this dish.

1. Dice & season the chicken.

2. Heat the olive oil in a frying pan and gently saute the onions & lemongrass for a few minutes until softened.

3. Add the chicken and cook for 4 minutes. Add the sugar, curry paste, lime juice, soy sauce & stock and cook for a further 2-4 minutes or until the chicken is cooked through.

4. Add the noodles & coconut milk and continue to cook until the dish is piping hot.

5. Divide into bowls and pile the watercress in a mound on top of each bowl.

Egg Molee

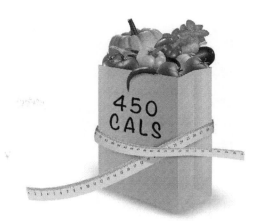

450 CALS

Ingredients — Serves 4

250g/9oz rice
2 garlic cloves, crushed
2 onions, chopped
250g/9oz peas
1 tbsp olive oil
2 tbsp tomato puree

1 tsp each turmeric, garam masala & ground ginger
250ml/1 cup low fat coconut milk
8 large free-range hard boiled eggs
Salt & pepper to taste

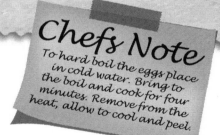

Chefs Note
To hard boil the eggs place in cold water. Bring to the boil and cook for four minutes. Remove from the heat, allow to cool and peel.

1. Place the rice in a pan of salted boiling water and cook until tender.

2. Gently saute the garlic, onions & peas in the olive oil for a few minutes until softened.

3. Stir through the tomato puree, dried spices & coconut milk until combined. Cut the eggs in half and place yolk side up, in the coconut milk. Gently cook until warmed through.

4. When everything is piping hot, drain the rice and spoon the curry on top.

5. Season and serve.

Spicy Lamb & Carrot Burger

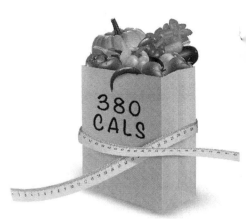

380 CALS

Ingredients　　Serves 4

500g/1lb 2oz lean lamb mince
2 carrots, peeled & grated
2 tbsp fresh breadcrumbs
2 large free-range eggs
2 garlic cloves, crushed
1 tsp English mustard

1 tsp cumin
2 large plum tomatoes, sliced
75g/3oz watercress
4 wholemeal bread rolls
Low cal cooking oil spray
Salt & pepper to taste

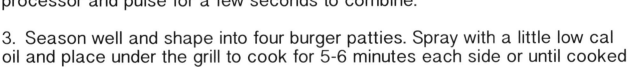

Chefs Note

This is great served with ketchup and/or a dollop of fat free Greek yogurt.

1. Preheat the grill.

2. Put the lamb mince, carrots, breadcrumbs, eggs, garlic, mustard & cumin in a food processor and pulse for a few seconds to combine.

3. Season well and shape into four burger patties. Spray with a little low cal oil and place under the grill to cook for 5-6 minutes each side or until cooked through.

4. Split open the rolls and when the burgers are cooked through place inside each roll.

5. Lay the sliced tomatoes on top of the burger along with the watercress.

6. Season and serve.

Lemon & Olive Penne

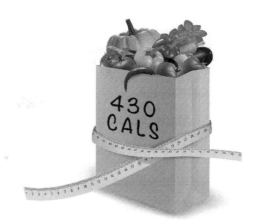

430 CALS

Ingredients
Serves 4

300g/11oz dried penne
1 tbsp olive oil
1 onion, sliced
2 garlic cloves, crushed
4 tbsp pitted black olives, sliced

1 tbsp balsamic vinegar
6 tbsp lemon juice
4 tbsp freshly chopped basil
200g/7oz low fat mozzarella cheese, cubed
Salt & pepper to taste

Chefs Note
Make sure you serve this dish when it is still nice and hot so that the mozzarella cheese remains melted.

1. Cook the penne in a pan of salted boiling water until tender.

2. Meanwhile heat the olive oil in a high-sided frying pan and gently saute the onions & garlic for 3-4 minutes. Add the olives, balsamic vinegar & lemon juice and cook until everything is tender and piping hot.

3. Drain the cooked penne and add to the frying pan along with the cubed mozzarella cheese. Stir through until the cheese melts.

4. Season and serve.

Creamy Parma Pasta

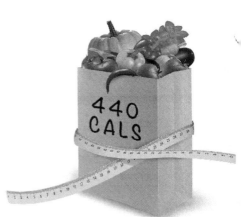

440 CALS

Ingredients   Serves 4

1 tbsp olive oil
1 onion, sliced
200g/7oz peas
6 slices Parma ham, chopped
120ml/½ cup low fat crème fraiche

300g/11oz dried fusilli
4 tbsp freshly chopped flat leaf parsley
1 tbsp grated Parmesan cheese
Salt & pepper to taste

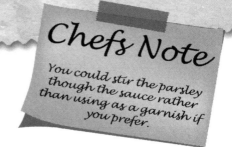

Chefs Note

You could stir the parsley though the sauce rather than using as a garnish if you prefer.

1. Cook the fusilli and peas in a pan of salted boiling water until tender.

2. Meanwhile heat the olive oil in a high-sided frying pan and gently saute the onions for a few minutes. When the onions are softened remove from the pan, increase the heat and add the chopped Parma ham. Cook until crispy, reduce the heat and return the onions to the pan along with the creme fraiche.

3. Drain the cooked pasta and add to the frying pan along with the Parmesan cheese.

4. Toss well and serve with the chopped parsley on top.

Asian Chicken Salad

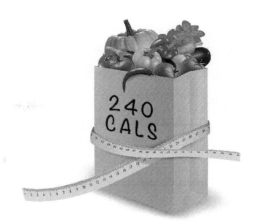

240 CALS

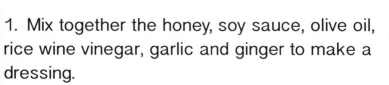

Ingredients — Serves 4

1 tbsp each runny honey, soy sauce, olive oil & freshly grated ginger
2 tbsp rice wine vinegar
2 garlic cloves, crushed
500g/1lb 2oz cooked chicken breast
½ red chilli, deseeded & finely chopped
1 cucumber, sliced into batons

2 carrots, thinly sliced into ribbons
1 bunch spring onions, thinly sliced lengthways
1 large romaine lettuces shredded
4 tbsp freshly chopped coriander
Salt & pepper to taste

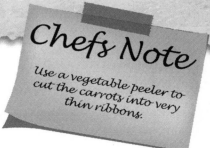

Chefs Note

Use a vegetable peeler to cut the carrots into very thin ribbons.

1. Mix together the honey, soy sauce, olive oil, rice wine vinegar, garlic and ginger to make a dressing.

2. Shred the cooked chicken. Place in a large bowl with the chilli, cucumber, carrots, spring onions and dressing. Combine well.

3. Arrange the shredded lettuce on four plates and pile the dressed chicken and vegetables on top.

4. Sprinkle with chopped coriander & serve.

Chicken & Broccoli Linguine

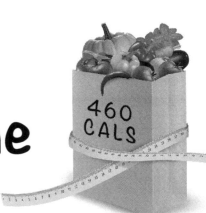

460 CALS

Ingredients   Serves 4

1 tbsp olive oil
2 garlic cloves, crushed
200g/7oz purple sprouting broccoli, roughly chopped
1 onion, sliced
400g/14oz skinless chicken breast, diced

300g/11oz linguine
1 tbsp tomato puree
250ml/1 cup tomato passata
100g/7oz rocket
Salt & pepper to taste

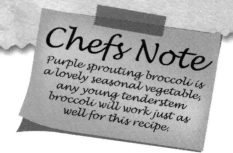

Chefs Note
Purple sprouting broccoli is a lovely seasonal vegetable; any young tenderstem broccoli will work just as well for this recipe.

1. Gently saute the garlic, broccoli, onions and chicken together in the olive oil for a few minutes in a high sided frying pan.

2. Meanwhile cook the linguine in a pan of salted boiling water until tender.

3. While the pasta is cooking add the tomato puree & passata to the frying pan and continue to cook until the chicken is cooked through and the broccoli is tender.

4. Drain the cooked linguine and add to the pan. Stir well and, when everything is combined, quickly toss through the rocket.

5. Balance the seasoning and serve immediately.

Scallop Sauce Spaghetti

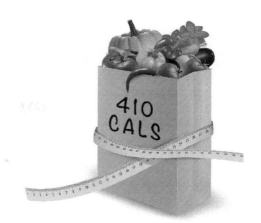

410 CALS

Ingredients
Serves 4

1 tbsp olive oil
1 onion, sliced
300g/11oz spaghetti
300g/11oz fresh, prepared scallops
60ml/¼ cup chicken stock
1 tbsp tomato puree

120ml/½ cup low fat crème fraiche
4 tbsp freshly chopped basil
Salt & pepper to taste

1. Cook the spaghetti in a pan of salted boiling water until tender.

Chefs Note
Reserve a little of the basil to use as a garnish if you wish.

2. Meanwhile gently heat the olive oil in a high-sided frying pan and saute the onion for 3-4 minutes whilst the pasta cooks. When the onions are softened add the scallops, chicken stock, tomato puree, creme fraiche & basil.

3. Cook for 5 minutes or until everything is cooked through. Place the contents of the pan in a blender to make a smooth sauce (add a little boiling water to loosen the sauce if needed).

4. Drain the pasta and toss well with the smooth scallop sauce.

5. Season and serve.

Salmon & Spanish Rice

400 CALS

Ingredients   Serves 4

250g/9oz rice
400g/14oz skinless salmon fillets
2 tbsp lemon juice
1 tbsp olive oil
1 onion, sliced
2 garlic cloves, crushed

2 large beef tomatoes, roughly chopped
100g/3½oz chorizo, finely chopped
1 tsp paprika
150g/5oz spinach
Salt & pepper to taste

Chefs Note
You could pan fry the salmon if you prefer by slicing into strips and adding to the sauté pan along with the chorizo.

1. Preheat the grill.

2. Place the rice in a pan of salted boiling water and cook until tender.

3. Brush the salmon fillets with lemon juice & a little olive oil and place under the grill.

4. Cook for 9-12 minutes (or longer if needed) until the salmon is cooked through and flakes easily.

5. Meanwhile gently saute the onions, garlic, chopped tomatoes, chorizo & paprika in a large high sided frying pan until everything softens and combines.

6. Flake the cooked salmon and tip it into the saute pan along with the drained rice and spinach. Stir well until the spinach wilts.

7. Season and serve.

Nepali Tuna Supper

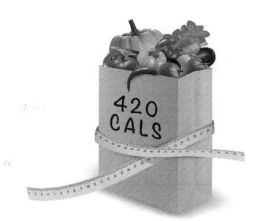

420 CALS

Ingredients
Serves 4

250g/9oz rice
1 tbsp olive oil
2 onions, sliced
2 garlic cloves, crushed
1 tbsp freshly grated ginger
1 tbsp curry powder

1 tsp ground coriander
1 red chilli, deseeded & finely sliced
500g/1lb 2oz tinned tuna steak, drained
Salt & pepper to taste

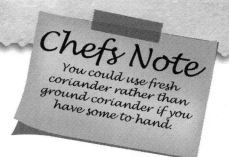

Chefs Note
You could use fresh coriander rather than ground coriander if you have some to hand.

1. Place the rice in a pan of salted boiling water and cook until tender.

2. Gently saute the onions and garlic in the olive oil for a 6-8 minutes until softened.

3. Add the ginger, curry powder, coriander, chilli and tuna steak and cook until piping hot (add a splash of water to the pan if needed)

4. When everything is piping hot tip the drained rice into the pan and combine well with the tuna and onions.

Venison Kebabs & Yoghurt

390 CALS

Ingredients   Serves 4

250g/9oz rice
6 venison sausages
1 tsp each ground cumin & turmeric
200g/7oz ripe cherry tomatoes
Low cal cooking oil spray

6 tbsp fat free Greek yoghurt
½ cucumber, finely chopped
2 tsp mint sauce
8 kebab skewers
Salt & pepper to taste

Chefs Note

If you use wooden skewers you will need to pre-soak them in water so that they don't burn.

1. Preheat the grill.

2. Place the rice in a pan of salted boiling water and cook until tender.

3. Skin the sausages and put in a food processor with the cumin and turmeric. Whizz for a few seconds to combine. Remove from the food processor and use your hands to shape into small kebab balls.

4. Place the venison balls and tomatoes in turn on the skewers and spray with a little oil.

5. Place the skewers under the grill and cook for 7-10 minutes or until cooked through.

6. Mix together the yoghurt, cucumber & mint to make a raita.

7. Divide the drained rice into bowls and serve with the cooked skewers on top and the minted raita on the side.

Lime & Thyme Squid Noodles

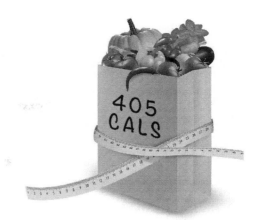

405 CALS

Ingredients   Serves 4

500g/1lb 2oz fresh thin squid rings
3 tbsp olive oil
2 garlic cloves, crushed
2 tbsp freshly chopped thyme
500g/1lb 2oz straight-to-wok medium noodles

200g/7oz peas
120ml/½ cup chicken stock
6 tbsp lime juice
Lime wedges to serve
Salt & pepper to taste

1. Season the squid well.

2. Mix together one tablespoon of olive oil, the garlic cloves & fresh thyme to make a dressing. Combine this with the squid rings and put to one side.

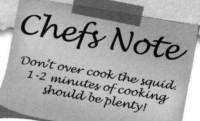

Chefs Note

Don't over cook the squid. 1-2 minutes of cooking should be plenty!

3. Cook the noodles and peas in the chicken stock in a saucepan until the stock reduces.

4. Mix together the lime juice and the remaining two tablespoons of olive oil.

5. Place the squid rings in a hot frying pan and cook for approximately 30 seconds each side, or until cooked through. Combine the fried squid, noodles & peas together along with the lime juice & olive oil.

6. Toss well, season and serve.

Mustard Haddock Chowder

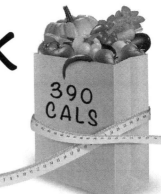

390 CALS

Ingredients   Serves 4

150g/5oz rice
1 tbsp olive oil
2 garlic cloves, crushed
1 onion, sliced
2 carrots, diced
150g/5oz potatoes, diced
1 tsp turmeric
1 tsp English mustard
500ml/2 cups semi skimmed milk
400g/14oz boneless, skinless smoked haddock fillets, cubed
4 tbsp freshly chopped flat leaf parsley
Salt & pepper to taste

Chefs Note

This is a really hearty chowder. You can make it go a little further by adding additional milk.

1. Place the rice in a pan of salted boiling water and cook until tender.

2. Gently saute the garlic, onions, carrots & potatoes for a few minutes until softened.

3. Add the turmeric, mustard, milk & haddock. Cover and leave to gently poach for 8-10 minutes or until the fish is cooked through and the vegetables are tender.

4. Add the drained rice to the milk pan.

5. Combine well, season and serve with parsley sprinkled over the top.

Watercress Gnocchi

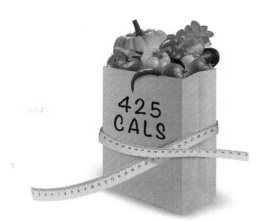

425 CALS

Ingredients
Serves 4

4 tbsp olive oil
1 tsp crushed garlic
1 onion, sliced

700g/1lb 9oz gnocchi
400g/14oz watercress
Salt & pepper to taste

1. Gently saute the garlic and onions in the olive oil for a few minutes

2. Whilst the onions are softening place the gnocchi in a pan of salted boiling water.

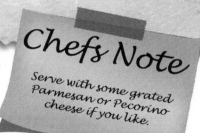

Chefs Note

Serve with some grated Parmesan or Pecorino cheese if you like.

3. Cook for 2-3 minutes or until the gnocchi begins to float to the top.

4. Meanwhile plunge the watercress into a fresh pan of boiling water and blanch for one minute. Drain and refresh immediately with cold water.

5. As soon as the gnocchi is cooked, drain and place in the frying pan with everything else.

6. Turn the heat up and move the gnocchi around for a few minutes to coat each dumpling in the oil and garlic and combine with the wilted watercress.

7. Check the seasoning and serve.

Jamaican Chicken Salad

340 CALS

Ingredients   Serves 4

500g/1lb 2oz skinless chicken breast
2 tsp crushed chilli flakes,
4 tbsp lime juice
1 tsp mixed spice
1 tbsp olive oil
1 onion, sliced

6 large plum tomatoes, roughly chopped
1 red pepper, deseeded & sliced
300g/11oz mixed salad leaves
Salt & pepper to taste

Chefs Note

This dish is good served with some fat free natural yoghurt to balance the heat of chilli.

1. Season the chicken and slice into thin strips.

2. Mix together the chilli flakes, lime juice, mixed spice and olive oil in a bowl to make a dressing. Add the chicken slices to the bowl and combine well.

3. Gently saute the dressed chicken, onions, tomatoes and peppers in the pan (add a little more oil if needed).

4. When the chicken is cooked through arrange on a bed of mixed salad leaves to serve.

Sweet & Spicy Steak Salad

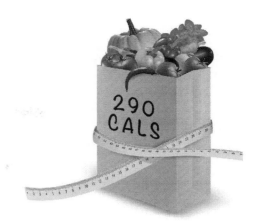

290 CALS

Ingredients   Serves 4

500g/1lb 2oz sirloin steak
2 tbsp olive oil
2 tsp runny honey
1 tbsp ketchup
1 tbsp soy sauce
3 tbsp lime juice

½ tsp crushed chilli flakes
4 large plum tomatoes, chopped
300g/11oz mixed spinach and rocket leaves
1 red onion, finely sliced
Salt & pepper to taste

Chefs Note

Adjust the cooking time depending on how you wish your steak to be cooked.

1. Trim any fat off the steak and lightly brush with a little of the olive oil. Season and slice into strips before putting a frying pan on a high heat.

2. Place the steak strips in the smoking-hot pan and cook for 1-2 minutes . Reduce the heat and add the rest of the olive oil, honey, ketchup, soy sauce, lime juice and chilli flakes.

3. Combine really well and cook for a minute or two longer.

4. Arrange the chopped tomatoes, salad leaves and red onion onto plates and place the sliced steak strips on top.

5. Season and serve.

Lemon & Oregano Tuna Steaks

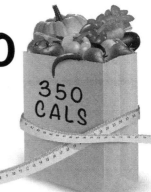

350 CALS

Ingredients   Serves 4

1 garlic clove, crushed
4 tbsp olive oil
2 tbsp lemon juice
4 tbsp freshly chopped oregano
4 fresh tuna steaks, each weighing 150g/5oz
200g/7oz cherry tomatoes, halved

1 red onion, sliced
150g/5oz watercress
Salt & pepper to taste

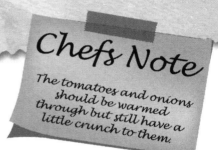

Chefs Note

The tomatoes and onions should be warmed through but still have a little crunch to them.

1. Mix together the garlic, olive oil, lemon juice & oregano in a bowl to make a dressing. Use a little of the dressing to brush on either side of the tuna steak. Place the halved tomatoes and sliced onions in the bowl with the rest of the dressing and coat well.

2. Put the tomatoes and red onions in a pan and saute for 2-4 minutes. Mix together the garlic, olive oil, lemon juice & oregano in a bowl to make a dressing. Use a little of the dressing to brush on either side of the tuna steak. Place the halved tomatoes and sliced onions in the bowl with the rest of the dressing and coat well.

3. Put the tomatoes and red onions in a pan and saute for 2-4 minutes. Whilst the tomatoes are cooking, place the tuna steak under a preheated medium grill and cook for 2-3 minutes each side or until the tuna is cooked to your liking.

4. Remove the tuna from the grill and serve with the onions and tomatoes piled on top and the watercress on the side.

Pea & Parmesan Risotto

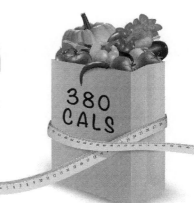

380 CALS

Ingredients   Serves 4

2 tbsp olive oil
1 garlic clove, crushed
1 onion, sliced
1 celery stalk, finely chopped
300g/11oz Arborio risotto

1lt/4 cups vegetable stock/broth
400g/7oz peas
1 tbsp fresh grated Parmesan cheese
Salt & pepper to taste

1. Heat the olive oil and gently saute the garlic, onion & celery for a few minutes until softened.

2. Add the risotto rice to the pan and stir well to coat each grain in olive oil. Add a ladle of stock and simmer until the stock is absorbed. Continue cooking the risotto adding a ladle of stock each time and allowing the rice to absorb the stock until adding the next ladle. Continue cooking for about 15 minutes or until the rice is tender. Add more stock if needed and continue the process until tender.

3. Meanwhile add the peas to boiling water and cook for 4-5 minutes or until tender. Add the drained peas to the pan and stir through the grated Parmesan cheese.

4. Season & serve.

Chefs Note
Risotto is traditionally made using white wine. Try substituting ¼ of the stock with wine if you like!

Greek Chicken Kebabs

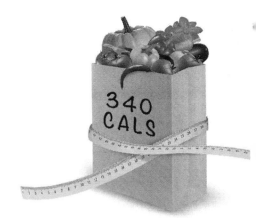

340 CALS

Ingredients   Serves 4

2 garlic cloves, crushed
1 tbsp olive oil
2 tsp dried oregano
3 tbsp lemon juice
500g/1lb 2oz skinless chicken breasts, cubed
200g/7oz rice

1lt/4 cups chicken stock
Salt & pepper to taste
Metal skewers

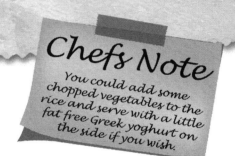

Chefs Note
You could add some chopped vegetables to the rice and serve with a little fat free Greek yoghurt on the side if you wish.

1. Preheat the grill to a medium/high heat.

2. Mix together the garlic, olive oil, oregano &
lemon juice in a bowl. Season the chicken and add to the bowl. Combine well
and skewer each piece to make four large chicken kebabs.

3. Place under the grill and cook for 6-8 minutes each side or until the
chicken is cooked through and piping hot.

4. Meanwhile cook the rice in the chicken stock until tender.

5. Remove the kebabs from the grill, season and serve with the drained rice.

Cavalfiori Risotto

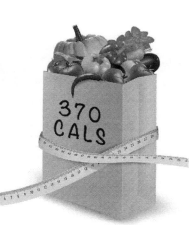

370 CALS

Ingredients

Serves 4

1 large cauliflower head
2 tbsp olive oil
2 garlic cloves, crushed
1 onion, sliced
1 celery stalk, finely chopped

300g/11oz Arborio risotto
1lt/4 cups vegetable stock/broth
4 tbsp freshly chopped flat leaf parsley
Salt & pepper to taste

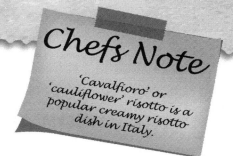

Chefs Note

'Cavalfioro' or 'cauliflower' risotto is a popular creamy risotto dish in Italy.

1. Break up the cauliflower head into florets and place in a food processor. Pulse until the cauliflower turns into rice sized grains.

2. Heat the olive oil and gently saute the onion, celery and garlic for a few minutes until softened. Add the risotto rice to the pan and stir well to coat each grain in olive oil. Add a ladle of stock and simmer until the stock is absorbed. Add the cauliflower to the pan. Continue cooking the risotto adding a ladle of stock each time and allowing the rice to absorb the stock until adding the next ladle. This should take about 15-20 minutes. Add more stock if needed and continue to cook until tender.

3. Season and serve with chopped parsley.

Fennel & Chickpea Chicken

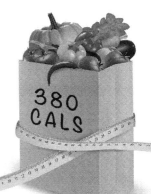

380 CALS

Ingredients Serves 4

1 tbsp olive oil
1 onion, sliced
1 celery stalk, finely chopped
2 carrots, diced
1 fennel bulb, finely sliced
1 tsp fennel seeds, crushed

3 garlic cloves, crushed
300g/11oz tinned chickpeas, drained
500g/1lb 2oz skinless chicken breasts, thickly sliced
120ml/½ cup chicken stock
Salt & pepper to taste

Chefs Note
You could serve this as a thick broth: add more stock and pulse for a few seconds in a blender or food processor.

1. Gently saute the onion, celery, carrots, fennel, fennel seeds & garlic in the olive oil for a few minutes until softened.

2. Add the chickpeas, chicken & stock and leave to gently simmer for 10-15 minutes or until the chicken is cooked through, the stock has reduced and the carrots are tender.

3. Season and serve.

Minted Fish Couscous

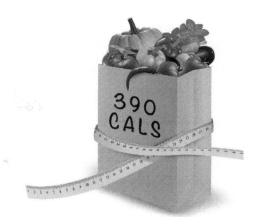

390 CALS

Ingredients Serves 4

400g/14oz skinless, boneless white fillets

2 garlic cloves, crushed

1 tbsp olive oil

2 tbsp lemon juice

1 large bunch fresh mint, finely chopped

4 large ripe beef tomatoes, thickly sliced

370ml/1½ cups chicken stock

200g/7oz couscous

Salt & pepper to taste

1. Preheat the grill to a medium/high heat.

2. Mix together the garlic, olive oil, lemon juice & mint and brush on either side of the fish fillets and tomato slices.

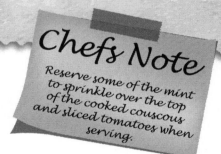

Chefs Note

Reserve some of the mint to sprinkle over the top of the cooked couscous and sliced tomatoes when serving.

3. Place the fish and tomato slices under the grill and cook for 2-3 minutes each side or until the fish is cooked through and the tomatoes are tender.

4. Meanwhile place the couscous in a pan with the hot stock. Bring the pan to the boil, remove from the heat, cover and leave to stand for 3-4 minutes or until all the stock is absorbed and the couscous is tender.

5. Fluff the couscous with a fork. Flake the fish and combine with the couscous.

6. Season & serve in shallow bowls with the grilled tomatoes on top.

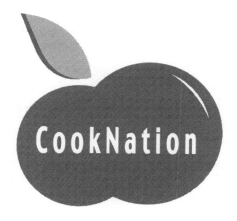

Other CookNation Titles

You may also be interested in other 'skinny' titles in the CookNation series.

You can find all the following great titles by searching under 'CookNation'.

Review

If you enjoyed 'The Skinny Low Calorie Recipe Book' we'd really appreciate your feedback. Reviews help others decide if this is the right book for them so a moment of your time would be appreciated. Thank you.

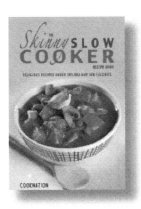

The Skinny Slow Cooker Recipe Book

Delicious Recipes Under 300, 400 And 500 Calories.

Paperback / eBook

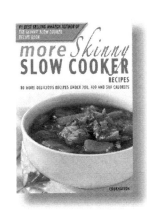

More Skinny Slow Cooker Recipes

75 More Delicious Recipes Under 300, 400 & 500 Calories.

Paperback / eBook

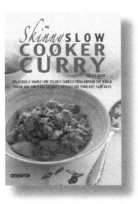

The Skinny Slow Cooker Curry Recipe Book

Low Calorie Curries From Around The World

Paperback / eBook

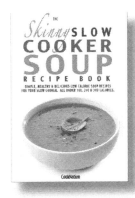

The Skinny Slow Cooker Soup Recipe Book

Simple, Healthy & Delicious Low Calorie Soup Recipes For Your Slow Cooker. All Under 100, 200 & 300 Calories.

Paperback / eBook

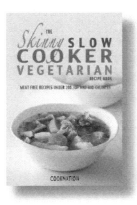

The Skinny Slow Cooker Vegetarian Recipe Book

40 Delicious Recipes Under 200, 300 And 400 Calories.

Paperback / eBook

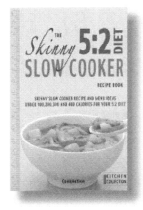

The Skinny 5:2 Slow Cooker Recipe Book

Skinny Slow Cooker Recipe And Menu Ideas Under 100, 200, 300 & 400 Calories For Your 5:2 Diet.

Paperback / eBook

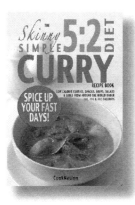

The Skinny 5:2 Curry Recipe Book

Spice Up Your Fast Days With Simple Low Calorie Curries, Snacks, Soups, Salads & Sides Under 200, 300 & 400 Calories

Paperback / eBook

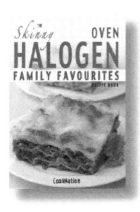

The Skinny Halogen Oven Family Favourites Recipe Book

Healthy, Low Calorie Family Meal-Time Halogen Oven Recipes Under 300, 400 and 500 Calories

Paperback / eBook

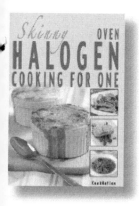

Skinny Halogen Oven Cooking For One

Single Serving, Healthy, Low Calorie Halogen Oven Recipes Under 200, 300 and 400 Calories

Paperback / eBook

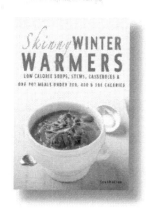

Skinny Winter Warmers Recipe Book

Soups, Stews, Casseroles & One Pot Meals Under 300, 400 & 500 Calories.

Paperback / eBook

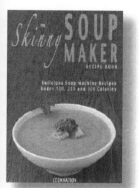

The Skinny Soup Maker Recipe Book

Delicious Low Calorie, Healthy and Simple Soup Recipes Under 100, 200 and 300 Calories. Perfect For Any Diet and Weight Loss Plan.

Paperback / eBook

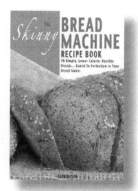

The Skinny Bread Machine Recipe Book

70 Simple, Lower Calorie, Healthy Breads...Baked To Perfection In Your Bread Maker.

Paperback / eBook

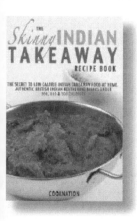

The Skinny Indian Takeaway Recipe Book

Authentic British Indian Restaurant Dishes Under 300, 400 And 500 Calories. The Secret To Low Calorie Indian Takeaway Food At Home

Paperback / eBook

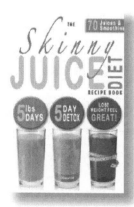

The Skinny Juice Diet Recipe Book

5lbs, 5 Days. The Ultimate Kick-Start Diet and Detox Plan to Lose Weight & Feel Great!

Paperback / eBook

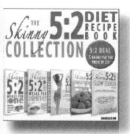

The Skinny 5:2 Diet Recipe Book Collection

All The 5:2 Fast Diet Recipes You'll Ever Need. All Under 100, 200, 300, 400 And 500 Calories

Available only on eBook

eBook

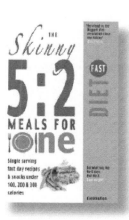

The Skinny 5:2 Fast Diet Meals For One

Single Serving Fast Day Recipes & Snacks Under 100, 200 & 300 Calories

Paperback / eBook

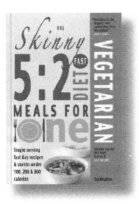

The Skinny 5:2 Fast Diet Vegetarian Meals For One

Single Serving Fast Day Recipes & Snacks Under 100, 200 & 300 Calories

Paperback / eBook

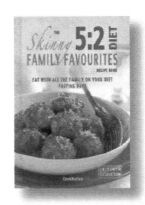

The Skinny 5:2 Fast Diet Family Favourites Recipe Book

Eat With All The Family On Your Diet Fasting Days

Paperback / eBook

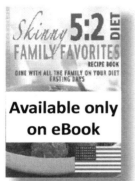

The Skinny 5:2 Fast Diet Family Favorites Recipe Book *U.S.A. EDITION*

Dine With All The Family On Your Diet Fasting Days

Paperback / eBook

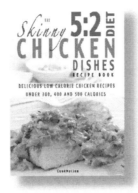

The Skinny 5:2 Diet Chicken Dishes Recipe Book

Delicious Low Calorie Chicken Dishes Under 300, 400 & 500 Calories

Paperback / eBook

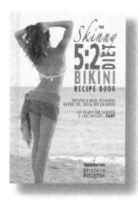

The Skinny 5:2 Bikini Diet Recipe Book

Recipes & Meal Planners Under 100, 200 & 300 Calories. Get Ready For Summer & Lose Weight...FAST!

Paperback / eBook

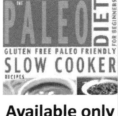
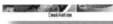

The Paleo Diet For Beginners Slow Cooker Recipe Book

Gluten Free, Everyday Essential Slow Cooker Paleo Recipes For Beginners

eBook

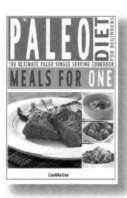

The Paleo Diet For Beginners Meals For One

The Ultimate Paleo Single Serving Cookbook

Paperback / eBook

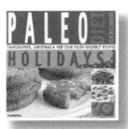

The Paleo Diet For Beginners Holidays

Thanksgiving, Christmas & New Year Paleo Friendly Recipes

eBook

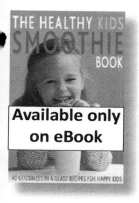

The Healthy Kids Smoothie Book

40 Delicious Goodness In A Glass Recipes for Happy Kids.

eBook

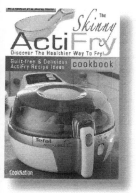

The Skinny ActiFry Cookbook

Guilt-free and Delicious ActiFry Recipe Ideas: Discover The Healthier Way to Fry!

Paperback / eBook

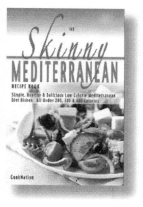

The Skinny Mediterranean Recipe Book

Simple, Healthy & Delicious Low Calorie Mediterranean Diet Dishes. All Under 200, 300 & 400 Calories.

Paperback / eBook

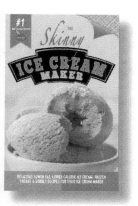

The Skinny Ice Cream Maker

Delicious Lower Fat, Lower Calorie Ice Cream, Frozen Yogurt & Sorbet Recipes For Your Ice Cream Maker

Paperback / eBook

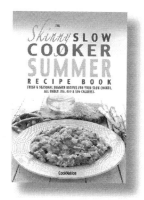

The Skinny Slow Cooker Summer Recipe Book

Fresh & Seasonal Summer Recipes For Your Slow Cooker. All Under 300, 400 And 500 Calories.

Paperback / eBook

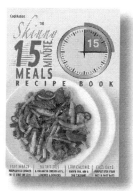

The Skinny 15 Minute Meals Recipe Book

Delicious, Nutritious & Super-Fast Meals in 15 Minutes Or Less. All Under 300, 400 & 500 Calories.

Paperback / eBook

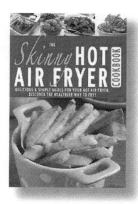

The Skinny Hot Air Fryer Cookbook

Delicious & Simple Meals For Your Hot Air Fryer: Discover The Healthier Way To Fry.

Paperback / eBook